The Complete
Diabetes Cookbook
& Meal Plan
For the
NEWLY DIAGNOSED

Alina Cobb

Disclaimer

The information provided in this book, "The Complete Diabetic Cookbook & Meal Plan for the Newly Diagnosed" is for educational and informational purposes only. It is not intended as a substitute for professional medical advice or treatment. Always seek the advice of your physician or other qualified healthcare provider with any questions regarding a medical condition.

While we have made every effort to ensure the accuracy and completeness of the content, we do not guarantee the reliability, suitability, or effectiveness of the recipes, suggestions, or dietary guidelines presented herein. The author, publisher, and contributors are not liable for any personal injury, damage, or loss arising from the use of the information presented in this book. Readers are responsible for their own health and should consult with a healthcare professional before making any dietary or lifestyle changes. The recipes and meal plans in this book are intended to promote healthy diabetic management and well-being, but individual results may vary.

It's important to consult with a qualified healthcare professional or nutritionist before making significant changes to your diet or lifestyle, especially if you have existing health conditions, allergies, or dietary restrictions.

The recipes and dietary recommendations in this book are based on general principles of nutrition, diabetes management, and healthy eating. Individual nutritional needs may vary, and what works well for one person may not be suitable for another.

We disclaim any liability for any loss, injury, or damage incurred as a result of the use or misuse of the information provided in this book. Readers are encouraged to use their own judgment and discretion when applying the content to their personal dietary and health practices.

By using this book, you agree that you are responsible for your own health decisions and understand that the information provided is not a substitute for professional medical advice or treatment. Always seek the advice of a qualified healthcare provider with any questions or concerns you may have regarding your health or dietary needs.

To Bob, for your unwavering support and constant encouragement. Your belief in me and your steadfast presence have been my rock during this journey. Thank you for always being there, for your kind words, and for inspiring me to keep going, even when times were tough. This book would not have been possible without you.

CONTENTS

Introduction **10**

PART ONE: For The Newly Diagnosed 11

Chapter 1: Now That You Are Diagnosed! 12

- What Does It Mean to Have Diabetes?................................14
- Why Do We Eat More Sugar Than Before?..........................15
- Signs and Symptoms of Diabetes.....................................15
- Key Questions for Newly Diagnosed Patients.....................17
- 30 Common Myths About Diabetes....................................19

Chapter 2: Nutrition and Diabetes 22

- Making Smart Nutrient Choices..23
- Taming the Beast of Cravings..24
- Notable Nutrients in Some Popular Vegetables..................25
- How Much Should I Eat?..26
- Plate Method for Meal Planning.......................................27

Chapter 3: Healthy Kitchen for Diabetes Management 29

- Food Options for Diabetic Friendly Meals..........................32

PART TWO: The Meal Plan 33

Chapter 4: The Four-Week Meal Plan 34

- Week 1: Establishing Healthy Habits.................................36
  - Diabetic meal plan..37
  - Grocery shopping list 38
- Week 2: Exploring Variety...39
  - Diabetic meal plan..40
  - Grocery shopping list..41
- Week 3: Enhancing Nutrition...42
  - Diabetic meal plan..43
  - Grocery shopping list..44
- Week 4: Mastering Your New Lifestyle..............................45
  - Diabetic meal plan..46
  - Grocery shopping list..47

PART THREE: The Recipes 48

Chapter 5: Breakfast Recipes 49

- Spinach and Feta Scramble 50
- Avocado and Egg Toast 50
- Greek Yogurt with Nuts and Seeds 51
- Tofu Scramble with Veggies 51
- Smoked Salmon and Avocado Plate 52
- Veggie-Stuffed Omelet 52
- Cottage Cheese and Veggie Bowl 53
- Mushroom and Spinach Breakfast Wrap 53
- Zucchini Fritters 54
- Turkey and Avocado Breakfast Sandwich 54
- Cauliflower Rice and Egg Bowl 55
- Chia Seed Pudding with Nuts 55
- Avocado & Chickpea Breakfast Salad 56
- Salmon and Spinach Frittata 56
- Quinoa Breakfast Bowl 57
- Lentil and Veggie Stir-Fry 57
- Egg and Avocado Breakfast Bowl 58
- Smoked Salmon and Avocado Toast 58
- Egg and Veggie Breakfast Muffins 59
- Almond Flour Pancakes with Greek Yogurt 59

Chapter 6: Lunch Recipes 60

- Spinach and Feta Stuffed Peppers 61
- Baked Salmon with Asparagus 61
- Tuna and Avocado Salad 62
- Chickpea and Vegetable Stir-Fry 62
- Grilled Chicken and Avocado Salad 63
- Quinoa and Black Bean Salad 63
- Turkey and Spinach Wrap 64
- Lentil and Vegetable Soup 64
- Chickpea and Spinach Curry 65
- Turkey and Vegetable Lettuce Wraps 65
- Cauliflower Rice and Shrimp Stir-Fry 66
- Chicken and Broccoli Stir-Fry 66
- Lentil and Vegetable Stew 67
- Tofu and Vegetable Stir-Fry 67
- Turkey and Avocado Wrap 68
- Zucchini Noodles with Pesto and Chicken 68

Chapter 7: Dinner Recipes 69

- Baked Salmon with Avocado Salsa 70
- Grilled Chicken with Quinoa and Spinach 70
- Baked Cod with Lemon and Asparagus 71
- Beef and Vegetable Skewers 71
- Shrimp and Vegetable Stir-Fry 72
- Turkey Meatballs with Zucchini Noodles 72

- Chicken and Vegetable Curry...73
- Tofu and Vegetable Stir-Fry..73
- Baked Chicken with Brussels Sprouts...74
- Lentil and Vegetable Stew...74
- Stuffed Bell Peppers with Ground Turkey...75
- Grilled Shrimp Tacos with Avocado...75
- Eggplant Parmesan...76
- Turkey and Spinach Stuffed Portobello Mushrooms...76
- Lemon Herb Grilled Chicken..77
- Spaghetti Squash with Tomato and Basil..77
- Salmon with Asparagus and Lemon...78
- Chicken and Broccoli Stir-Fry...78
- Quinoa and Black Bean Stuffed Zucchini..79
- Baked Cod with Tomatoes and Olives..79

Chapter 8: Desserts Recipes 80

- Avocado Chocolate Mousse..81
- Chia Seed Pudding...81
- Greek Yogurt Parfait..82
- Almond Flour Cookies..82
- Berry and Spinach Smoothie..83
- Coconut and Almond Energy Balls...83
- Blueberry Almond Crisp..84
- Coconut and Almond Energy Balls...84

Chapter 9: Snacks and Appetizers Recipes 85

- Apple and Walnut Salad..86
- Baked Pears with Cinnamon...86
- Blueberry Almond Crisp..87
- Pumpkin Protein Bars..87
- Avocado Deviled Eggs..88
- Cucumber and Hummus Bites...88
- Greek Yogurt and Veggie Dip...89
- Turkey and Cheese Roll-Ups..89
- Spiced Nuts...90
- Lentil and Veggie Lettuce Wraps..90
- Caprese Skewers...91
- Spinach & Feta Stuffed Mushrooms..91
- Edamame with Sea Salt...92
- Guacamole with Bell Pepper Slices...92

Chapter 10: Salads and Sides Recipes 93

- Grilled Chicken and Spinach Salad...94
- Lentil and Tomato Salad...94
- Quinoa and Kale Salad...95
- Tuna and Avocado Salad..95
- Greek Yogurt and Cucumber Salad...96
- Chickpea and Spinach Salad..96
- Shrimp and Avocado Salad..97
- Turkey and Berry Salad..97
- Bean and Corn Salad...98
- Egg and Asparagus Salad...98

Chapter 11: Vegetarian Options Recipes 99

- Roasted Brussels Sprouts with Almonds........100
- Spinach and Mushroom Sauté........100
- Cauliflower Rice with Herbs........101
- Baked Zucchini Fries........101
- Roasted Asparagus with Lemon and Parmesan........102
- Garlic Green Beans........102
- Cucumber and Tomato Salad........103
- Baked Eggplant with Tahini........103
- Roasted Carrot and Lentil Salad........104
- Stuffed Bell Peppers with Quinoa........104

Chapter 12: Chicken & Turkey Options Recipes 105

- Lemon Herb Chicken Breast........106
- Avocado Chicken Salad........106
- Spinach and Chicken Stuffed Peppers........107
- Chicken and Lentil Soup........107
- Baked Chicken with Brussels Sprouts........108
- Chicken and Vegetable Skewers........108
- Chicken Lettuce Wraps........109
- Turkey and Avocado Wrap........109

Chapter 13: Beef, Pork & Lamb Recipes 110

- Beef and Broccoli Stir-Fry........111
- Pork Tenderloin with Spinach........111
- Lamb Chops with Roasted Vegetables........112
- Beef and Lentil Stew........112
- Lamb and Quinoa Salad........113
- Beef and Cauliflower Rice Bowl........113
- Pork and Cabbage Stir-Fry........114
- Lamb and Vegetable Kebabs........114
- Beef and Apple Skillet........115
- Pork and Apple Skillet........115

Chapter 14: Fish and Seafood Recipes 116

- Grilled Salmon with Avocado Salsa........117
- Shrimp and Vegetable Stir-Fry........117
- Baked Cod with Spinach & Tomatoes........118
- Tuna and Avocado Salad........118
- Garlic Butter Shrimp and Asparagus........119
- Seared Scallops with Spinach and Mushrooms........119
- Lemon Herb Baked Tilapia........120
- Salmon and Quinoa Salad........120
- Spicy Shrimp with Cauliflower Rice........121
- Lemon Garlic Butter Fish........121

Chapter 15: Soup Recipes **122**

- Chicken and Vegetable Soup...123
- Lentil and Spinach Soup...123
- Broccoli and Cauliflower Soup...124
- Turkey and Vegetable Soup..124
- Tomato and Basil Soup...125
- Butternut Squash Soup...125
- Mushroom and Barley Soup...126
- Split Pea Soup..126
- Cauliflower and Leek Soup...127
- Turkey Meatball Soup...127

Chapter 16: Smoothie Recipes **128**

- Berry Spinach Protein Smoothie..129
- Green Avocado Smoothie...129
- Peanut Butter Banana Smoothie..130
- Blueberry Almond Smoothie...130
- Tropical Green Smoothie..131
- Spinach and Kiwi Smoothie..131
- Cucumber Mint Smoothie...132
- Chocolate Peanut Butter Smoothie..132
- Strawberry Basil Smoothie...133
- Pumpkin Spice Smoothie...133

Conclusion **134**

Appendix **136**

- Appendix 1: The 2024 Dirty Dozen™ and Clean Fifteen™...................................136
- Appendix 2: Measurement Conversions 137
- Appendix 3: Carb Content of Foods...138
- Appendix 4: Recipe Index..140

Introduction

Imagine standing at the edge of a dense forest, feeling uncertain and maybe even a bit scared. The path ahead is unfamiliar, and you can't see where it leads. This is how many people feel when they are first diagnosed with diabetes. But what if I told you that beyond those trees lies a beautiful, thriving garden? The key to reaching that garden is knowledge, and that's exactly what this book aims to provide.

If you've just found out you have type 2 diabetes and you're feeling lost, overwhelmed, and unsure about what to do next, you're not alone. As a registered dietitian and diabetes educator for over ten years, I've seen how tough it can be to deal with this news. I've heard people share their anger, frustration, and sadness. But more importantly, I've helped them find the right tools and strategies to take control and make positive changes. I wrote this book to help others who might not have the chance to meet with me in person.

In PART ONE of the book, we'll demystify diabetes and help you understand what it truly means to have this condition. We'll explore why we consume more sugar than ever before, recognize the signs and symptoms of diabetes, and address the key questions that often arise after diagnosis. We'll debunk 30 common myths about diabetes, and equip you with vital information on nutrition and maintaining a healthy kitchen for diabetes management. This part is all about laying a strong foundation, giving you the confidence and clarity to navigate your new reality.

The PART TWO is a Meal Plan, where we start to build on that foundation, guiding you through a structured Four-Week Meal Plan. Each week is designed to introduce you to delicious, balanced meals that will help stabilize your blood sugar levels. With detailed grocery shopping lists and practical tips, you'll find meal planning and preparation easier than ever. This section is like your roadmap through the forest, showing you the way to that beautiful, thriving garden.

Finally, in PART THREE: The Recipes, we delve into a rich array of diabetic-friendly recipes. From hearty breakfasts to satisfying dinners, delectable desserts to wholesome snacks, this section is your treasure trove of culinary delights. Whether you're in the mood for vegetarian options, savory chicken and turkey dishes, succulent beef, pork, and lamb recipes, fresh fish and seafood, comforting soups, or refreshing smoothies, you'll find something to satisfy every craving.

Let's embark on this journey together. Remember, you are not alone. Each page of this book is crafted to support you, inspire you, and empower you to take control of your health. Embrace this new chapter with an open heart and mind. Your journey towards better health starts now, and with the right tools and mindset, you can transform your diagnosis into an opportunity for growth and wellness.

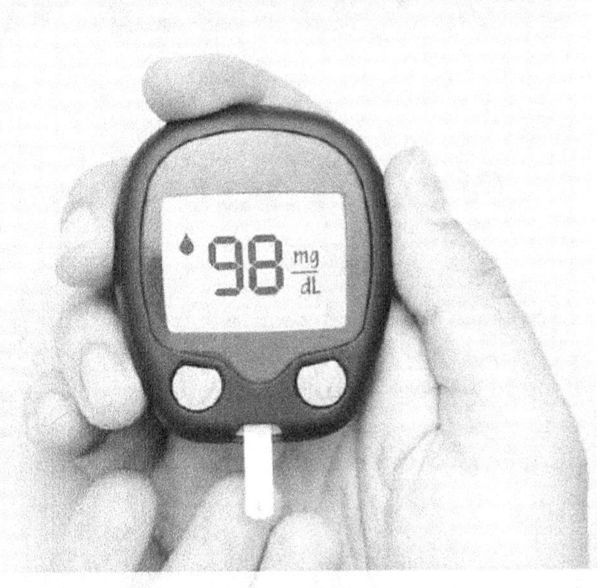

PART ONE:

FOR THE NEWLY DIAGNOSED

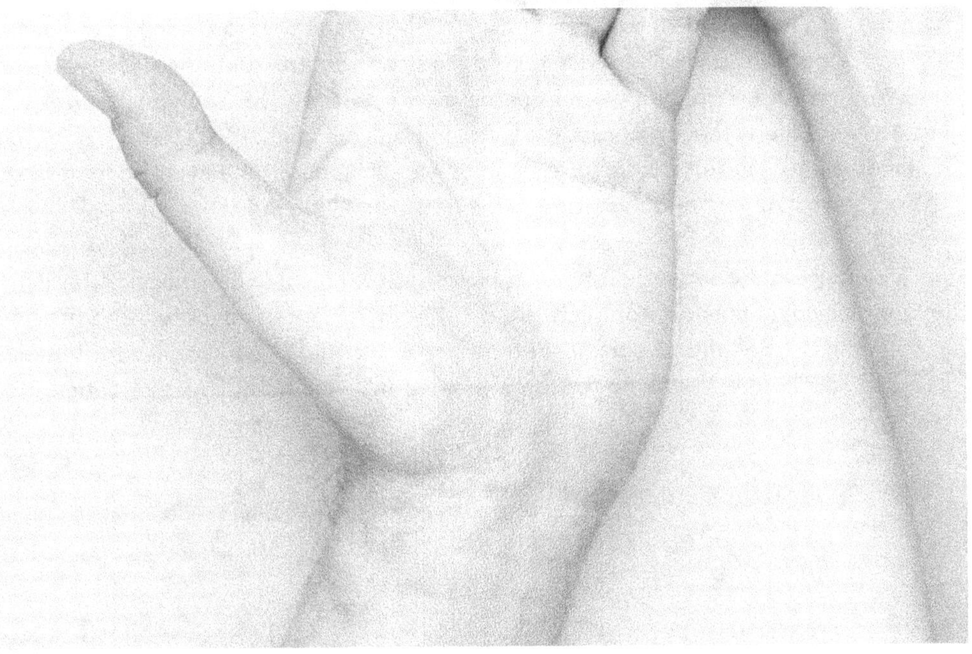

Now That You Are Diagnosed!

If you've just been diagnosed with type 2 diabetes and are feeling lost, overwhelmed, and unsure of your next steps, you're not alone. As a registered dietitian and diabetes educator with over a decade of experience, I've witnessed the emotional rollercoaster that often follows a diabetes diagnosis. I've heard clients express their anger, frustration, and sadness. But most importantly, I've guided them toward the resources and strategies they need to take control and make positive changes.

Hundreds of millions of people worldwide are living with diabetes, and many don't even know it. Often, it's an unpleasant surprise diagnosis when you visit the hospital or see your doctor for something else, only to hear the unwelcome news that you have diabetes. Almost everyone knows someone with diabetes—a friend or family member might have tearfully shared their bad news, or you've noticed they've made sudden, drastic lifestyle changes. Maybe you've even heard your own doctor say, "You have type 2 diabetes."

It's normal to feel like a victim, especially if diabetes seemed to come out of nowhere. It can feel like you're carrying a villain inside you that you can't control. But remember, while it's okay to feel this way, you also have the power to change your perspective. You can live well with diabetes and lead a great life without it constantly weighing on your mind. It will require some changes and a commitment to yourself, but you are the one who will benefit the most from these adjustments. Taking control of your health means you're the one calling the shots.

Unlike many other diseases, diabetes is manageable. You'll want a support team to help you on this journey, including your doctor, dietitian, nutritionist, diabetes educator, and pharmacist. Once you understand the benefits of certain methods, how to avoid pitfalls, and adapt to changes that improve your health, there's no reason why you can't live life on your own terms and be happy and healthy.

Managing diabetes might require medications to regulate your insulin. You may be able to reduce or even eliminate these over time, depending on your blood sugar levels. Keeping your blood sugar as close to your target as possible is crucial for preventing or delaying diabetes-related complications, which is often what scares us the most about this condition. We've all heard the horror stories.

I won't pretend this will be easy, but by regularly checking your blood sugar levels and making adjustments where you can, you'll soon see that diabetes isn't the monster you might have thought it was. Some people resist making the necessary changes, but you're different. By choosing this book, you've shown that you're ready to act and take charge of your life. In these pages, you'll learn how to make small adjustments to feel better, look better, manage your condition, and continue living a vibrant and adventurous life.

Whether you're dealing with type 1 diabetes (where your body doesn't produce enough insulin) or type 2 diabetes (where your body resists insulin), the core issue is too much sugar piling up in your blood. Left unchecked, this excess sugar can overwork your kidneys, causing it to spill into your urine. High blood sugar is destructive—it can break down tissues, potentially leading to blindness, kidney failure, strokes, and heart attacks. It also damages your nerves, resulting in numbness, tingling, and pain. Poor circulation from diabetes can cause wounds to heal slowly, sometimes leading to severe complications like amputations.

Diabetes rates have skyrocketed over the past 35 years, with over 38 million Americans now living with either type 1 or type 2 diabetes. Sharing these facts isn't to scare you but to empower you to make smarter choices and resist unhealthy temptations. These small, essential changes can stop the fear you felt at diagnosis from becoming your everyday reality.

The root cause of your cells struggling to absorb sugar for energy and growth is a substance that resists insulin: fat. The silver lining is that type 1 diabetes can be managed with insulin, and type 2 diabetes can be controlled with medications. However, the most effective and healthiest way to tackle type 2 diabetes is by embracing an active lifestyle and eating a nutritious diet.
You are in control of both!

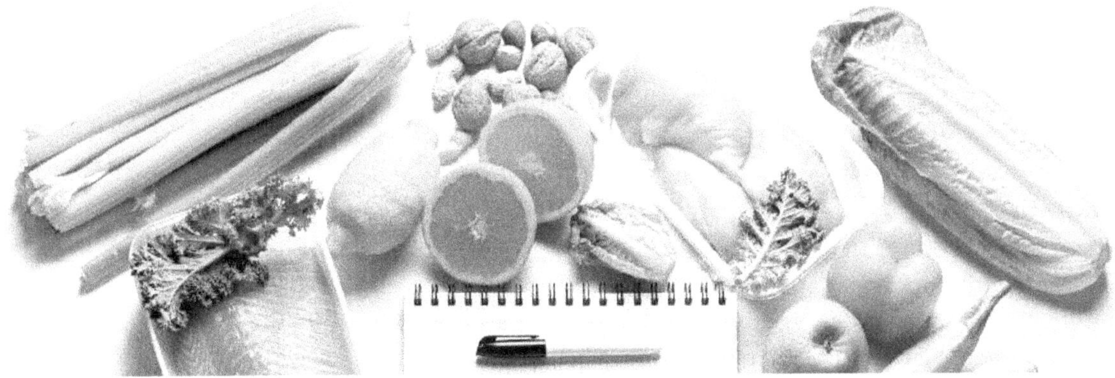

What Does It Mean to Have Diabetes?

Being diagnosed with type 2 diabetes can feel overwhelming and confusing. You might think you did something wrong, but that's not the case. It's not about blame or judgment. Plenty of people eat and drink the same things without developing diabetes. Often, the difference comes down to genetics. You might have inherited genes from your parents or grandparents that increase your risk for diabetes, but that doesn't mean you're doomed. Lifestyle choices play an even bigger role in managing and even preventing diabetes.

Understanding Diabetes

When your doctor tells you, "You have type 2 diabetes," it usually follows a series of blood tests showing higher-than-normal blood sugar levels. This means both your fasting blood sugar (when you wake up) and your post-meal blood sugar (two hours after eating) are elevated.

How Blood Sugar Works

Everyone has sugar in their blood, known as glucose, which fuels every cell in your body. Your brain, in particular, relies solely on glucose for energy. Glucose comes from the carbohydrates in foods like bread, potatoes, rice, pasta, and refined sugars.

After you eat, glucose is absorbed into your bloodstream, causing your blood sugar levels to rise. Normally, a fasting blood sugar level is about 90 mg/dL (5 mmol/L), and it's normal for it to rise by about two points after eating.

In response to this rise, your pancreas releases insulin. Insulin acts like a key, attaching to receptors on your cells and unlocking them so glucose can enter. Once inside, glucose is used to generate energy, bringing your blood sugar levels back down.

The Diabetes Difference

With diabetes, this cycle changes. Your fasting blood sugar is often higher than 90 mg/dL, and your post-meal levels rise more than they should. This imbalance can be managed with the right approach.

Taking Control

Managing diabetes starts with understanding how your body processes sugar and the impact of different foods and activities on your glucose levels. This book will guide you through the best nutrition and lifestyle practices to adopt. These habits are about more than just managing diabetes; they're about improving your overall health and vitality.

Why Do We Eat More Sugar Than Before?

In nature, we're meant to get glucose (sugar) from plants. Back then, plants had fiber along with sugar, which slowed down how fast our bodies absorbed the sugar. But today, most of the foods we eat are processed and have lots of sugar and starch, but no fiber. Fiber is often removed so these foods can stay fresh longer and be sold in stores.

When foods are processed, they lose their fiber and become sweeter. We love sweetness because our ancestors knew sweet things were safe to eat and gave them energy. Our brains release a chemical called dopamine when we eat something sweet, making us feel good. This is why we crave sugary foods.

Thousands of years ago, humans started making plants even sweeter through breeding. Eventually, we made table sugar from sugarcane, which became super popular. But getting sugar became linked to terrible things like slavery.

Today, sugar is everywhere, and we eat a lot more of it than before. Our brains love the taste, but too much sugar isn't good for us. It can cause health problems without us even knowing. So, while sugar makes us happy and gives us energy, too much of it can be harmful. We need to find a balance in how much sugar we eat for a healthy life.

Signs and Symptoms of Diabetes

Recognizing the signs and symptoms of diabetes is crucial for early diagnosis and effective management. The symptoms can vary depending on the type of diabetes and how elevated the blood sugar levels are. Here are the common signs and symptoms for both type 1 and type 2 diabetes:

Common Symptoms of Diabetes

1. Frequent Urination:
High blood sugar levels cause the kidneys to filter out excess glucose, leading to increased urine production and frequent urination.

2. Excessive Thirst:
The increased urine production leads to dehydration, causing excessive thirst and increased fluid intake.

3. Extreme Hunger:
Despite having high blood sugar levels, the cells are not receiving glucose, which can lead to increased hunger as the body tries to get the energy it needs.
 susceptibility to infections.

4. Unexplained Weight Loss:
In type 1 diabetes, the body starts to break down fat and muscle for energy because it can't use glucose properly, leading to weight loss. In type 2 diabetes, weight loss can also occur, though it's less common.

5. Fatigue:
 The lack of glucose in the cells leads to low energy levels and fatigue, making individuals feel tired and weak.

6. Blurred Vision:
High blood sugar levels can cause swelling in the lens of the eye, leading to blurred vision.

7. Slow-Healing Sores or Frequent Infections:
Elevated blood sugar levels can impair blood circulation and the immune system, leading to slow-healing wounds and increased susceptibility to infections.

Positive Changes Ahead

One of the most encouraging aspects of this journey is the positive change you'll experience. Many people who adopt these strategies report feeling better than they have in years. Improved energy levels, better mood, and healthier blood sugar levels are common outcomes. This transformation is not just about managing a condition but reclaiming your health and enjoying a higher quality of life.

Moving Forward

It's crucial to remember that every day is an opportunity to make choices that support your health. While the path may have its challenges, the knowledge and tools you'll gain from this book will empower you to navigate them with confidence. You'll learn how to organize your kitchen and pantry strategically, make nutritious meals, and understand the science behind your food choices.

Simple adjustments in your daily routine can lead to significant improvements in your blood sugar levels and overall health. Being diagnosed with diabetes is not the end of your health journey but the beginning of a new, informed chapter. With the right knowledge and habits, you can control your blood sugar levels effectively and avoid becoming part of any scary statistics. As you follow the guidance in this book, you'll likely find yourself feeling better than you have in years, enjoying normal, healthy blood sugar levels, and living a vibrant, balanced life.

Remember, taking control of your lifestyle can make a huge difference, no matter what your genes say.

Key Questions for The Newly Diagnosed

What exactly is diabetes, and how does it affect my body?
- Diabetes is a condition where your body struggles to control blood sugar levels. This happens because your body either doesn't produce enough insulin (a hormone that helps regulate blood sugar) or it can't use insulin properly. High blood sugar can lead to symptoms like thirst, frequent urination, and fatigue, and if not managed well, it can cause complications like heart disease, nerve damage, and vision problems.

What type of diabetes do I have, and how does it differ from other types?
- There are mainly two types of diabetes. Type 1 diabetes means your body doesn't produce insulin at all, so you need to take insulin injections. Type 2 diabetes means your body isn't using insulin effectively or isn't producing enough, and it's often managed with lifestyle changes and sometimes medication. It's important to know your type because treatment plans vary.

What should my target blood sugar range be, and why is it important?
- Your target blood sugar range will depend on your specific health needs and treatment goals. Generally, fasting blood sugar should be between 80-130 mg/dL, and after meals, it should be less than 180 mg/dL. Staying within this range helps prevent symptoms and reduces the risk of long-term complications like heart disease and nerve damage.

How can I monitor my blood sugar levels at home, and how often should I check them?
- You can monitor your blood sugar with a glucometer, a small device that measures the sugar level in a drop of blood. Your doctor will guide you on how often to check—often a few times a day depending on your treatment plan. Regular monitoring helps you see how well your management plan is working and lets you make adjustments as needed.

What foods should I avoid, and what should I include in my diet?
- Avoid sugary snacks, sugary drinks, and high-carb foods like white bread and pastries. Instead, focus on eating vegetables, whole grains, lean proteins, and healthy fats. Foods like leafy greens, nuts, and berries are great choices. These foods help keep your blood sugar steady and provide important nutrients.

How does physical activity affect my blood sugar levels, and what exercises are best for me?
- Regular physical activity helps your body use insulin more effectively and can lower blood sugar levels. Aim for at least 150 minutes of moderate exercise, like brisk walking or cycling, each week. Combining cardio with strength training (like lifting weights or yoga) is also beneficial for overall health and blood sugar control.

What are the signs of high and low blood sugar, and how should I handle them?

- High blood sugar can cause symptoms like excessive thirst, frequent urination, and blurred vision. Low blood sugar might make you feel shaky, dizzy, or hungry. For high blood sugar, drink plenty of water and follow your doctor's advice for insulin or medication. For low blood sugar, eat or drink something with fast-acting carbs, like fruit juice or glucose tablets.

Are there any medications I need to take, and what are their side effects?

- You might need medications to help control your blood sugar. Common ones include metformin, insulin, or other drugs that improve insulin sensitivity. Side effects vary by medication but can include nausea, weight gain, or low blood sugar. Your doctor will help you find the best option with the fewest side effects.

How do my medications work, and what should I know about taking them?

- Medications work by either increasing insulin production, improving your body's insulin sensitivity, or helping your body use sugar more efficiently. It's crucial to take them exactly as prescribed—never skip doses or change the amount without consulting your doctor. Consistency helps keep your blood sugar in check.

How does stress impact my diabetes, and what strategies can I use to manage it?

- Stress can raise blood sugar levels by triggering hormones that increase glucose production. To manage stress, try relaxation techniques like deep breathing, meditation, or exercise. Regular physical activity and a healthy diet also help keep stress levels in check and maintain stable blood sugar.

What long-term complications should I be aware of, and how can I prevent them?

- Long-term complications can include heart disease, nerve damage, kidney problems, and vision issues. Prevent them by managing your blood sugar levels well, keeping blood pressure and cholesterol in check, and getting regular check-ups. Good self-care and following your treatment plan are key.

How can I recognize and manage diabetic foot problems?

- Look for signs like cuts, blisters, or sores on your feet, and check them daily. Diabetes can cause numbness and poor circulation, making foot injuries worse. Keep your feet clean and dry, wear comfortable shoes, and see a podiatrist regularly to catch and address any issues early.

30 Common Myths About Diabetes

Myth: Only overweight people get diabetes.
Fact: Diabetes can affect people of all body types. While obesity is a risk factor, genetics and other factors play a role.

Myth: Diabetes is caused by eating too much sugar.
- Fact: Diabetes is related to how your body handles blood sugar, not just sugar intake. A balanced diet is important, but diabetes is influenced by multiple factors.

Myth: You can't eat carbohydrates if you have diabetes.
- Fact: Carbohydrates are an important part of a balanced diet. Managing portion sizes and choosing complex carbs can help control blood sugar levels.

Myth: People with diabetes can't eat fruit.
- Fact: Fruits are nutritious and can be part of a diabetes-friendly diet. The key is moderation and choosing fruits with lower glycemic indexes.

Myth: Insulin is only for people with Type 1 diabetes.
- Fact: Insulin is used in both Type 1 and Type 2 diabetes. People with Type 2 diabetes may need insulin if other treatments aren't sufficient.

Myth: You'll outgrow Type 1 diabetes.
- Fact: Type 1 diabetes is a lifelong condition. It requires ongoing management and does not go away.

Myth: Diabetes is always diagnosed in childhood or old age.
- Fact: Type 1 diabetes can occur at any age, and Type 2 diabetes is increasingly being diagnosed in younger people due to rising obesity rates.

Myth: You can stop taking diabetes medication if your blood sugar levels improve.
- Fact: Diabetes management often requires ongoing medication and lifestyle changes. Always consult your doctor before changing your treatment plan.

Myth: People with diabetes can't exercise.
- Fact: Regular exercise is beneficial for people with diabetes. It helps manage blood sugar levels and overall health.

Myth: You have to eat special "diabetic" foods.
- Fact: There is no need for special foods. A healthy, balanced diet that includes a variety of foods is best for managing diabetes.

Myth: Diabetes means you have to give up all your favorite foods.
- Fact: You can still enjoy your favorite foods in moderation. Portion control and balanced choices are key.

Myth: Diabetes only affects the elderly.
- Fact: While Type 2 diabetes is more common in older adults, it can occur at any age. Type 1 diabetes often begins in childhood or young adulthood.

Myth: People with diabetes will always lose weight.
- Fact: Weight loss is not a guaranteed outcome of diabetes. Some people may gain weight or have difficulty losing weight despite having diabetes.

Myth: You can tell if someone has diabetes just by looking at them.
- Fact: Diabetes is not always visible. People with diabetes can appear healthy and may not have obvious symptoms.

Myth: Diabetes is not a serious condition.
- Fact: Diabetes is a serious chronic condition that can lead to complications such as heart disease, kidney failure, and nerve damage if not properly managed.

Myth: Diabetics can't have any sweets or desserts.
- Fact: People with diabetes can enjoy sweets in moderation. It's important to account for them in your meal plan and balance them with other healthy foods.

Myth: Diabetes only affects blood sugar levels.
- Fact: Diabetes can impact various aspects of health, including cardiovascular health, kidney function, and nerve sensation.

Myth: Diabetic people can't have a healthy pregnancy.
- Fact: With proper management and medical care, people with diabetes can have healthy pregnancies. Monitoring blood sugar and working with healthcare providers is crucial.

Myth: Type 2 diabetes is not as serious as Type 1 diabetes.
- Fact: Both types of diabetes are serious and require effective management to prevent complications. Type 2 diabetes can also lead to significant health issues if not controlled.

Myth: You can't travel or enjoy vacations if you have diabetes.
- Fact: People with diabetes can travel and enjoy vacations. It's important to plan ahead, manage your medication, and follow your diabetes care routine while away.

Myth: Diabetes is a result of poor willpower or lack of self-control.
- Fact: Diabetes is a complex condition influenced by genetics, biology, and lifestyle factors. It is not a matter of willpower or self-discipline.

Myth: You have to test your blood sugar frequently to manage diabetes.
- Fact: The frequency of blood sugar testing depends on individual needs and treatment plans. Some people may need to test more often, while others may not need to test as frequently.

Myth: Natural remedies can cure diabetes.
- Fact: There is no cure for diabetes. While some natural remedies may help manage blood sugar levels, they should be used in conjunction with conventional medical treatments.

Myth: Diabetes only requires managing blood sugar levels.
- Fact: Managing diabetes involves more than just blood sugar control. It includes monitoring blood pressure, cholesterol levels, and overall lifestyle.

Myth: Diabetic complications are inevitable.
- Fact: Many complications can be prevented or delayed with proper diabetes management, including maintaining good blood sugar control and regular medical check-ups.

Myth: You should avoid all fats if you have diabetes.
- Fact: Healthy fats, like those from avocados, nuts, and olive oil, are important for a balanced diet. The focus should be on reducing unhealthy fats and including healthy fats in moderation.

Myth: If your blood sugar levels are normal, you don't need to worry about diabetes anymore.
- Fact: Diabetes requires ongoing management and monitoring. Normal blood sugar levels are a sign that your plan is working, but continued care is essential to prevent complications.

Myth: You can manage diabetes with diet alone.
- Fact: While diet is a crucial part of diabetes management, it often needs to be combined with medication, physical activity, and regular monitoring.

Myth: Diabetes only affects adults.
- Fact: Type 1 diabetes often develops in children and young adults, and Type 2 diabetes is increasingly being diagnosed in younger populations due to rising obesity rates.

Myth: Diabetes is the same for everyone.
- Fact: Diabetes management is individualized. Each person's treatment plan is tailored to their specific needs, lifestyle, and health conditions.

Nutrition and Diabetes

Understanding the essential nutrients and how they affect your body is crucial for managing diabetes. Let's break down the basics of carbohydrates, proteins, fats, and essential vitamins and minerals to see how they play a role in your health.

Carbohydrates

Carbohydrates often get a bad rap, but they are essential for providing energy to your body, especially your brain and muscles. When you eat carbs, your body breaks them down into glucose (sugar), which is then used for energy.

- **Types of Carbohydrates:** There are two main types of carbs: simple and complex. Simple carbs are found in sugary foods and drinks, and they can cause quick spikes in blood sugar levels. Complex carbs, like those found in whole grains, vegetables, and legumes, break down more slowly, leading to more stable blood sugar levels.
- **Fiber:** A type of complex carbohydrate found in fruits, vegetables, and whole grains. Fiber helps with digestion, keeps you feeling full, and stabilizes blood sugar levels.

Fats

Fats are another misunderstood nutrient. They are not just a source of energy but also essential for various bodily functions.
- **Healthy Fats:** These include unsaturated fats found in olive oil, avocados, nuts, and fish. They help with hormone production, vitamin absorption, and maintaining healthy cell membranes.
- **Unhealthy Fats:** Saturated and trans fats, found in fried foods, baked goods, and some animal products, can increase the risk of heart disease and should be limited.

Proteins

Proteins are the building blocks of life. They are vital for growth, repair, and maintenance of tissues in your body.
- **Sources of Protein:** Include lean meats, fish, eggs, dairy products, beans, and legumes. Incorporating a variety of protein sources in your diet ensures you get all the essential amino acids your body needs.
- **Role in Diabetes Management:** Protein helps stabilize blood sugar levels by slowing down the absorption of carbohydrates. It also keeps you feeling full longer, which can help with weight management.

Essential Vitamins and Minerals

Vitamins and minerals, also known as micronutrients, are essential for various bodily functions and overall health.

- **Vitamin D:** Helps regulate insulin sensitivity and is essential for bone health. You can get vitamin D from sunlight, fortified foods, and supplements.

- **Magnesium:** Plays a role in insulin metabolism and helps control blood sugar levels. Foods rich in magnesium include leafy greens, nuts, seeds, and whole grains.

- **Sodium:** While sodium is essential for fluid balance and nerve function, it's important to manage your intake. Too much sodium can lead to high blood pressure, which is a risk factor for diabetes complications. Opt for low-sodium options and limit processed foods.

- **Potassium:** Helps balance the effects of sodium and supports heart health. Potassium-rich foods include bananas, oranges, potatoes, and spinach.

- **Calcium:** Essential for bone health and proper function of your heart, muscles, and nerves. Dairy products, leafy greens, and fortified plant-based milks are good sources of calcium.

Making Smart Nutrient Choices

Balancing these nutrients in your diet is key to managing diabetes effectively. Here are some tips to help you make smart choices:

- **Prioritize Whole Foods:** Choose whole grains, fresh fruits, vegetables, lean proteins, and healthy fats over processed foods.
- **Read Labels:** Understanding nutrition labels can help you make better choices by revealing the amount of carbs, fats, and sodium in packaged foods.
- **Plan Balanced Meals:** Aim to include a mix of carbohydrates, proteins, and fats in each meal to help keep your blood sugar levels stable.

By understanding and managing your intake of these essential nutrients, you can take control of your health and effectively manage your diabetes. Remember, making small, informed changes can lead to significant improvements in your overall well-being.

Taming the Beast of Cravings

Ah, cravings—the notorious disruptors of even the most meticulously planned weeks. Understanding your body's nutritional needs can help you stay ahead of these urges and keep your diet on track. Below are some essential nutrients our bodies crave, which can often go overlooked during busy periods or festive seasons.

Nutrient Needs and Smart Swaps

Stock up on these healthy substitutes to satisfy your body's true needs when cravings strike. By consistently providing your body with nutritious alternatives, you'll not only curb immediate cravings but also reduce their frequency over time.

- Craving Sweets? Reach for fresh fruit like apples, berries, or a small piece of dark chocolate (75% cocoa or higher).
- Craving Salty Snacks? Opt for a handful of unsalted nuts, seeds, or air-popped popcorn.
- Craving Crunchy Foods? Try raw vegetables like carrots, bell peppers, or celery sticks with a bit of hummus.
- Craving Comfort Foods? Satisfy with a warm bowl of oatmeal topped with cinnamon and a few nuts or seeds.

By keeping these healthy options readily available, you'll teach your body to expect and be satisfied with nutritious food, effectively managing those pesky cravings.

You Crave	What You Need	Healthy Alternatives to Eat
Oily Foods	Calcium	Organic milk, cheese, leafy greens
Chocolate	Magnesium	Raw cacao, nuts, seeds, veggies, fruits
Bread, pasta & other carbs	Nitrogen	High protein foods, meat, fish, nuts, beans, chia seeds
Salty Foods	Chloride	Fatty fish, goat milk, radishes
Sugary foods	Sulphur	Cabbage, Cranberries, Cauliflower
	Carbon	Fresh fruit (berries, apples)
	Chromium	Chicken, Broccoli, grapes, cheese,
	Tryptophan	Sweet potato, Cheese, Raisins, Spinach
	Phosphorus	Veggies, Fish, Chicken, Eggs, Dairy, Nuts

Notable Nutrients in Some Popular Vegetables

Vegetable	Vitamins	Minerals	Phytonutrients
Spinach	Vitamins C, K, A, B6 and Folate	Manganese, Potassium, Magnesium, Calcium, Iron	Flavonoids, Carotenoids
Red Cabbage	Vitamins C, K, B6 and Folate	Manganese, Potassium	Glucosinolates, Flavonoids, Anthocyanins
Green Cabbage	Vitamins C, K, B6 and Folate	Manganese, Potassium	Glucosinolates, Flavonoids
Cauliflower	Vitamins C, K, B6, Folate and Pantothenic Acid	Manganese, Potassium	Glucosinolates, Flavonoids
Kale	Vitamins C, K, A, B6	Manganese, Potassium, Magnesium, Calcium, Iron	Glucosinolates, Flavonoids, Carotenoids
Broccoli	Vitamins C, K, A, B6 and Folate	Manganese, Potassium	Glucosinolates, Flavonoids, Carotenoids
Brussels Sprouts	Vitamins C, K, A, B6 and Folate	Manganese, Potassium	Glucosinolates, Flavonoids, Carotenoids
Romaine Lettuce	Vitamins C, K, A and Folate	Manganese, Potassium	Flavonoids, Carotenoids

How Much Should I Eat?

Finding the right balance of food is essential for maintaining steady blood sugar levels and overall health. This section will guide you through planning your meals to ensure you're eating the right amount of food in the right combinations. Your caloric intake should typically range between 2000 and 2800 calories per day, but it's crucial to consult with your doctor to tailor this figure to your specific needs, taking into account your age, activity level, and diabetes management strategy. Let's dive into how to plan your plate for optimal glucose control

Understanding Your Caloric Needs

Your daily caloric needs depend on several factors:

- **Age:** Your metabolism slows as you age, requiring fewer calories.
- **Activity Level:** More active individuals need more calories to fuel their bodies.
- **Diabetes Management:** Your specific diabetes treatment plan may affect your calorie needs.

Consult with your healthcare provider to determine your ideal caloric intake. Once you have this number, you can start planning your meals to fit within these guidelines.

Plate Method for Meal Planning

Plate planning is a powerful tool that can help you manage your blood sugar levels effectively. It involves carefully selecting and portioning different types of foods to ensure a balanced diet that supports your overall health and well-being. The Plate Method is a simple, effective way to visualize and manage your portions. Here's how to break down your plate:

1. **Half Your Plate: Non-Starchy Vegetables**
   - Fill half your plate with a variety of non-starchy vegetables like leafy greens, broccoli, peppers, and carrots. These are low in calories and carbohydrates, high in fiber, and packed with essential vitamins and minerals.
   - Benefits: They help fill you up without spiking your blood sugar and provide important nutrients for overall health.
2. **Quarter Your Plate: Lean Protein**
   - Allocate a quarter of your plate to lean protein sources such as chicken, turkey, fish, eggs, tofu, and legumes. Protein helps stabilize blood sugar levels and keeps you feeling full longer.
   - Benefits: Supports muscle maintenance and repair, and helps manage hunger and blood sugar levels.
3. **Quarter Your Plate: Whole Grains and Starchy Vegetables**
   - The remaining quarter should be dedicated to whole grains and starchy vegetables like brown rice, quinoa, whole-wheat pasta, sweet potatoes, and corn. These provide necessary carbohydrates for energy but should be consumed in moderation.
   - Benefits: Whole grains offer more fiber and nutrients compared to refined grains, helping to maintain steady blood sugar levels.

Plate Method for Meal Planning

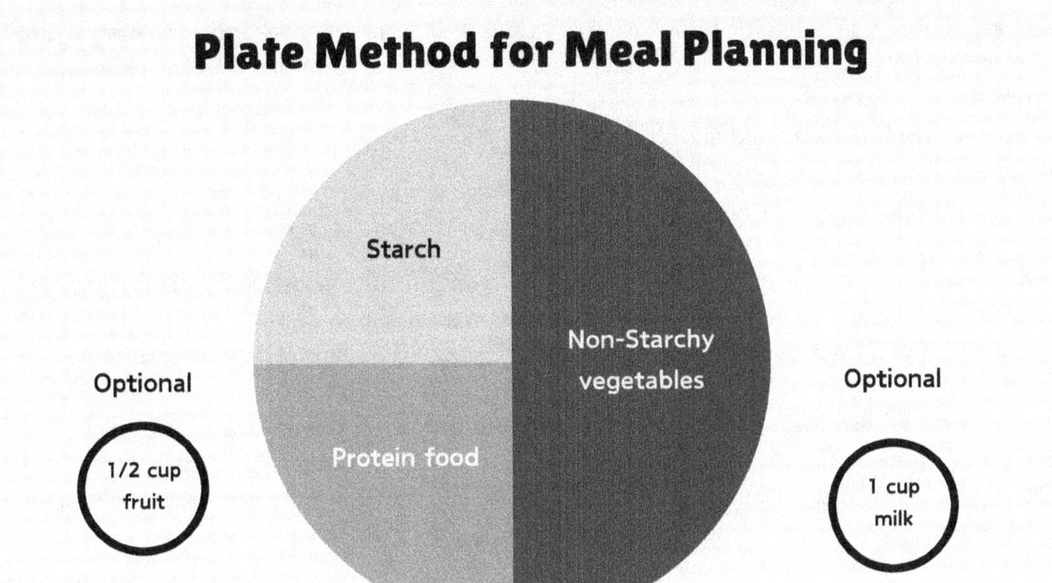

Healthy Fats
- Don't forget to include healthy fats in your diet. Add a small amount of healthy fats like avocado, nuts, seeds, and olive oil to your meals.
- Benefits: Fats are essential for nutrient absorption and hormone production, and they help keep you satiated.

Portion Control

Understanding portion sizes is crucial for maintaining glucose control:
- Vegetables: Unlimited non-starchy vegetables.
- Protein: Aim for about 3-4 ounces of lean protein per meal (about the size of a deck of cards).
- Carbohydrates: Keep starchy vegetables and whole grains to about 1/2 cup per meal.
- Fats: Limit to about 1-2 tablespoons of healthy fats per meal.

Tips for Balanced Meals
- **Breakfast:** Start your day with a balanced meal that includes protein, such as eggs or Greek yogurt, paired with whole grains like oatmeal and a serving of fruit.
- **Lunch:** A salad with a variety of vegetables, lean protein like grilled chicken, and a small portion of whole grains like quinoa.
- **Dinner:** Grilled fish with roasted vegetables and a side of brown rice or a sweet potato.

- **Snacks:** Snacks can help maintain your energy levels and prevent overeating at meals. Opt for nutrient-dense snacks that include a mix of carbohydrates, proteins, and fats. Some smart snack ideas include:
  - A small apple with a handful of almonds.
  - Greek yogurt with berries.
  - Carrot sticks with hummus.

- **Hydration:** Staying hydrated is just as important as your food choices. Water helps regulate body temperature, transport nutrients, and remove waste. Aim to drink at least 8 glasses of water a day, and consider incorporating other low-calorie beverages like herbal teas.

- **Monitor and Adjust:** Regularly monitor your blood sugar levels to see how your body responds to different foods and meal combinations. Keeping a food diary can be helpful in tracking your intake and identifying patterns. Adjust your portion sizes and food choices based on your blood sugar readings and how you feel.

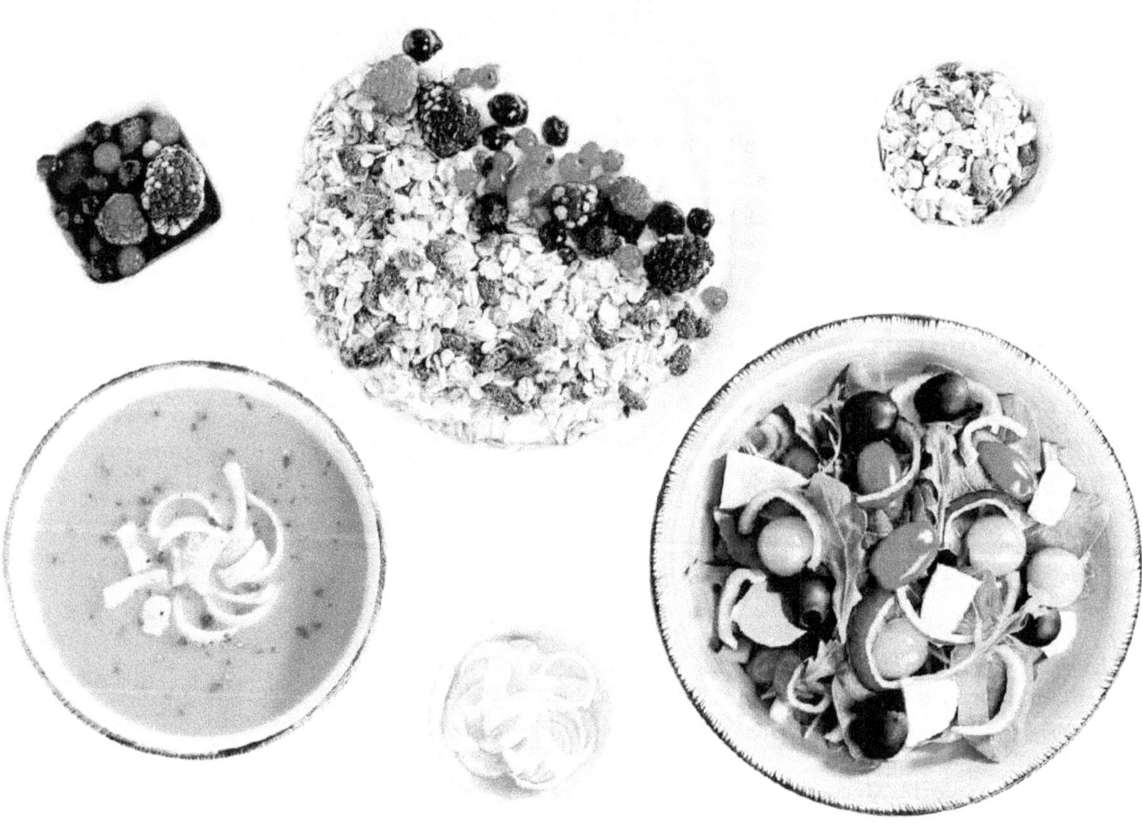

Chapter Three

Healthy Kitchen for Diabetes Management

Creating a healthy and nutritious diet plan for yourself isn't rocket science, but sometimes it can seem daunting, especially when your stomach is growling and there's nothing in the kitchen to fix. Rebuilding your kitchen does not mean you need to go out and buy a lot of fancy, expensive equipment. It simply means setting you up for success by stocking it with the things that will enable you to make easy meals every day. That means the pantry items you'll use most often and the necessary tools to organize, prep, and cook your food. Having what you need on hand will make meal planning less time-consuming and will ensure that you're easily able to follow your diabetes nutrition guidelines every day—which will create the long-term results you are looking for.

Here's a list of items to keep on hand as back-ups when the weekend sneaks up on you, or the unprepared work-week leaves you tired with the cupboard bare.

Whole Grains and Legumes

- Quinoa: A versatile grain that is high in protein and fiber.
- Brown Rice: A nutritious alternative to white rice with more fiber and nutrients.
- Oats (Rolled and Quick): Great for breakfast or baking, oats are high in fiber and can help stabilize blood sugar.
- Whole Wheat Flour: For baking and cooking.
- Lentils and Beans: These are excellent sources of protein, fiber, and essential nutrients.

Protein-Rich Foods

- Canned Tuna, Salmon, and Haddock: Convenient sources of protein and omega-3 fatty acids.
- Wild Salmon, Swordfish, and Mackerel: High in protein and healthy fats.
- Eggs: Versatile and nutrient-dense, eggs can be used in many dishes.
- Greek Yogurt: High in protein and probiotics, it can be used in sweet and savory dishes.
- Almond Butter and Natural Peanut Butter: Great for snacks or adding to meals.
- Nuts and Seeds (Almonds, Walnuts, Cashews, Pepitas, Chia Seeds, Flaxseed, Hemp Seeds): High in protein and healthy fats.

Fresh and Frozen Vegetables

- Leafy Greens (Spinach, Kale, Arugula): Rich in vitamins and can be used in salads, smoothies, or sautés.
- Bell Peppers: High in vitamin C and can be eaten raw or cooked.
- Broccoli and Cauliflower: High in fiber and can be roasted, steamed, or added to stir-fries.
- Frozen Mixed Vegetables: A quick and easy way to add variety to meals.
- Red Onions, Carrots, and Avocados: Essential for various dishes, providing vitamins and healthy fats.
- Garlic and Ginger: Both have numerous health benefits and can enhance the flavor of your meals.

Fruits

- Berries (Strawberries, Blueberries, Raspberries, Loganberries): Low in sugar and high in antioxidants.
- Apples: High in fiber and easy to grab on the go.
- Citrus Fruits: Oranges, grapefruits, and lemons provide vitamin C and can enhance the flavor of many dishes.
- Frozen Fruit: Great for smoothies or a quick, healthy dessert.

Healthy Fats

- Olive Oil: A heart-healthy oil for cooking and dressings.
- Coconut Oil: Another good option for cooking, with a different flavor profile.
- Avocado Oil: High in healthy fats and suitable for high-heat cooking.

Herbs and Spices

- Cinnamon and Turmeric: Known for their potential to help regulate blood sugar levels and anti-inflammatory properties.
- Garlic Powder, Onion Powder, Ginger (Ground), and Paprika: Essential for flavoring various dishes.
- Basil, Oregano, Thyme, Coriander, Cumin, Curry Powder, Italian Seasoning Blend: Fresh or dried, these herbs and spices add flavor without added salt or sugar.
- Bay Leaves, Cloves, Chili Powder, Fennel Seeds: Enhance the complexity of your meals.

Dairy and Dairy Alternatives

- Milk or Plant-Based Milks (Almond, Soy, Oat): Options for cooking and drinking.
- Cheese: Opt for lower-fat varieties or those made from goat's or sheep's milk.
- Cottage Cheese: High in protein and versatile for both sweet and savory dishes.

Pantry Essentials

- Low-Sodium Broth (Chicken, Beef, or Vegetable): For soups and stews.
- Canned Tomatoes: Use them in sauces, soups, or stews.
- Apple Cider Vinegar, Balsamic Vinegar, Red Wine Vinegar, Rice Wine Vinegar: For dressings and marinades.
- Mustard, Soy Sauce (Low Sodium, Gluten-Free), Worcestershire Sauce: Flavorful additions without added sugar.
- Nonstick Cooking Spray (Olive, Coconut, or Canola Oil): For healthy cooking without excessive fats.
- Baking Powder, Cocoa Powder (Unsweetened), Cornstarch: For baking and cooking needs.
- Pure Maple Syrup, Honey: Natural sweeteners for various recipes.

Healthy Snacks

- Air-Popped Popcorn: A whole grain snack that can be seasoned to taste.
- Hummus: A protein-rich dip for vegetables or whole-grain crackers.
- Dark Chocolate (75% Plus): Choose varieties with at least 75% cocoa for a lower-sugar treat.

The key to a well-stocked pantry is organization. While it may sound like simple advice, clearing out the clutter and stocking up on staples will ensure you always know what foods you have available and that you always have the basics on hand to whip up a quick meal any day of the week. I recommend having several shelves, clear containers, bags, and baskets in your pantry so that you can easily see your groceries—no digging and shuffling required. Try to commit one or two minutes a day to maintaining your pantry's organization, as well. This will provide the additional bonus of helping you cut back on food waste.

By keeping these staples in your kitchen, you can create a variety of balanced, nutritious meals and snacks that support diabetes management. Planning and preparing in advance can help ensure you always have healthy options available, making it easier to stick to your dietary goals even on the busiest days.

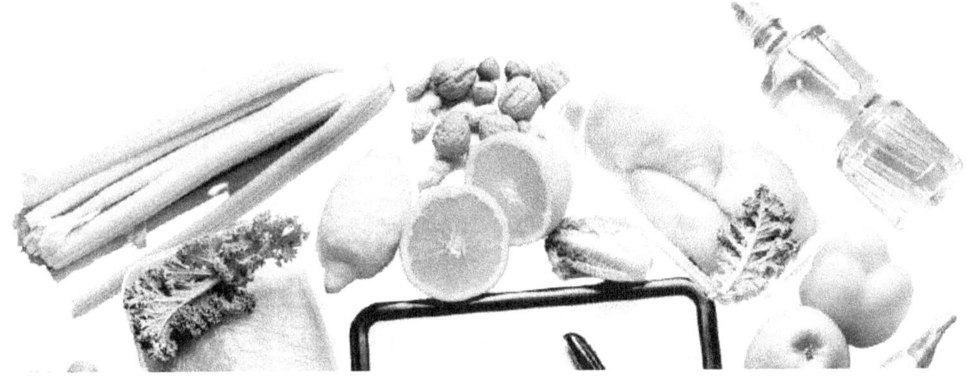

Food Options for Diabetic Friendly Meals

Starchy foods	Protein-rich foods	Non-starchy vegetables
• Sweet potatoes • Quinoa • Brown rice • Wild rice • Barley • Bulgur • Steel-cut oats • Rolled oats • Buckwheat • Farro • Spelt • Millet • Amaranth • Sorghum • Freekeh • Whole grain bread • Whole grain pasta • Lentils • Chickpeas • Black beans • Kidney beans • Navy beans • Pinto beans • Green peas • Corn • Butternut squash • Acorn squash • Pumpkin • Plantains • Parsnips	• Skinless chicken breast • Turkey breast • Lean cuts of beef (e.g.sirloin or tenderloin) • Lean cuts of pork (e.g. loin or tenderloin) • Fish (e.g. salmon, tuna, and cod) • Shellfish (e.g. shrimp, crab, and lobster) • Eggs • Egg whites • Greek yogurt (unsweetened) • Cottage cheese (low-fat) • Tofu • Tempeh • Edamame • Lentils • Chickpeas • Black beans • Kidney beans • Navy beans • Quinoa • Chia seeds • Flaxseeds • Hemp seeds • Pumpkin seeds • Sunflower seeds • Almonds • Walnuts • Peanuts • Pistachios • Cashews • Low-fat cheese (e.g. mozzarella or ricotta)	• Spinach • Kale • Broccoli • Cauliflower • Brussels sprouts • Asparagus • Bell peppers • Zucchini • Cucumber • Green beans • Lettuce • Cabbage • Swiss chard • Collard greens • Bok choy • Radishes • Arugula • Celery • Mushrooms • Tomatoes • Eggplant • Onions • Leeks • Garlic • Okra • Turnips • Fennel • Endive • Artichokes • Snow peas

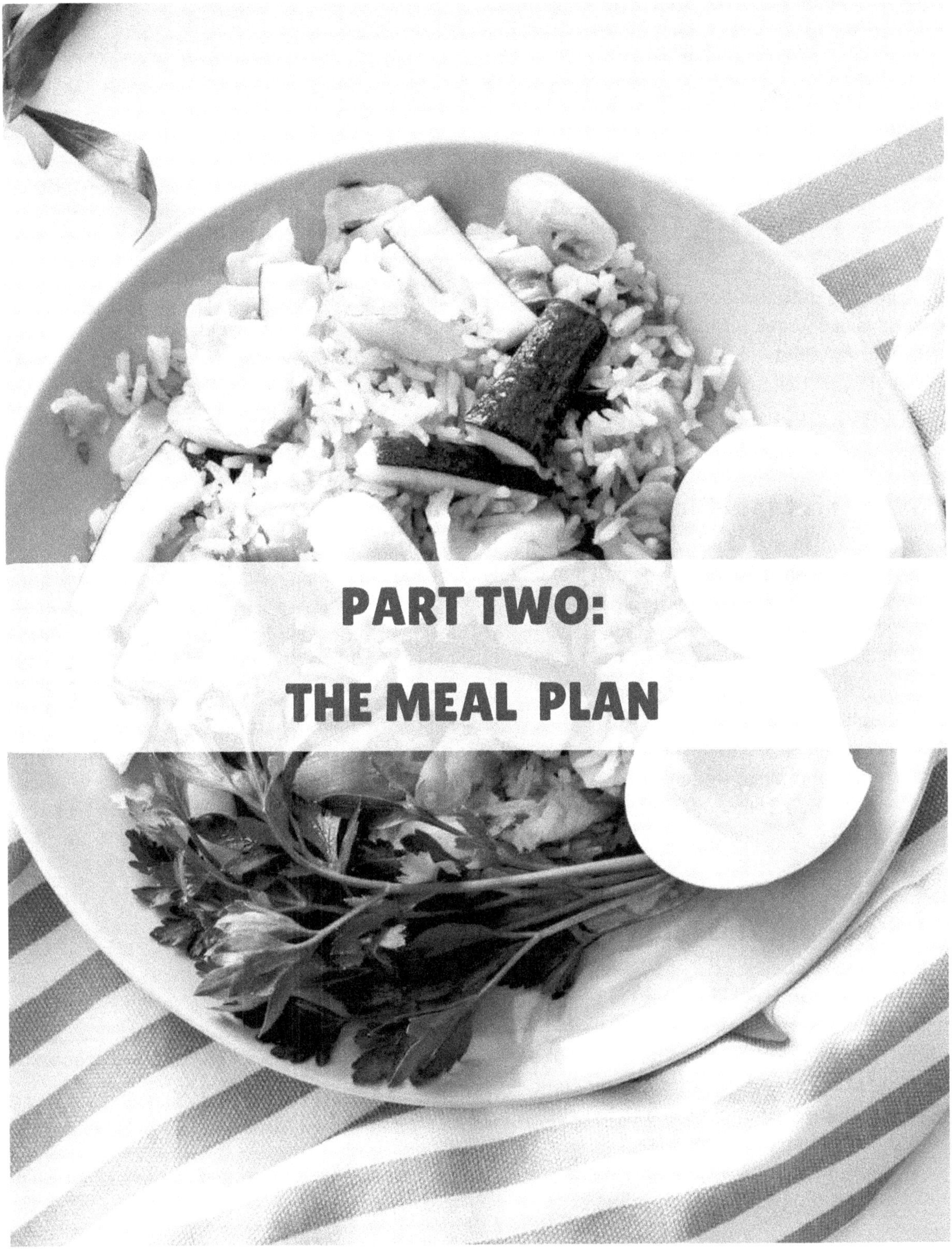

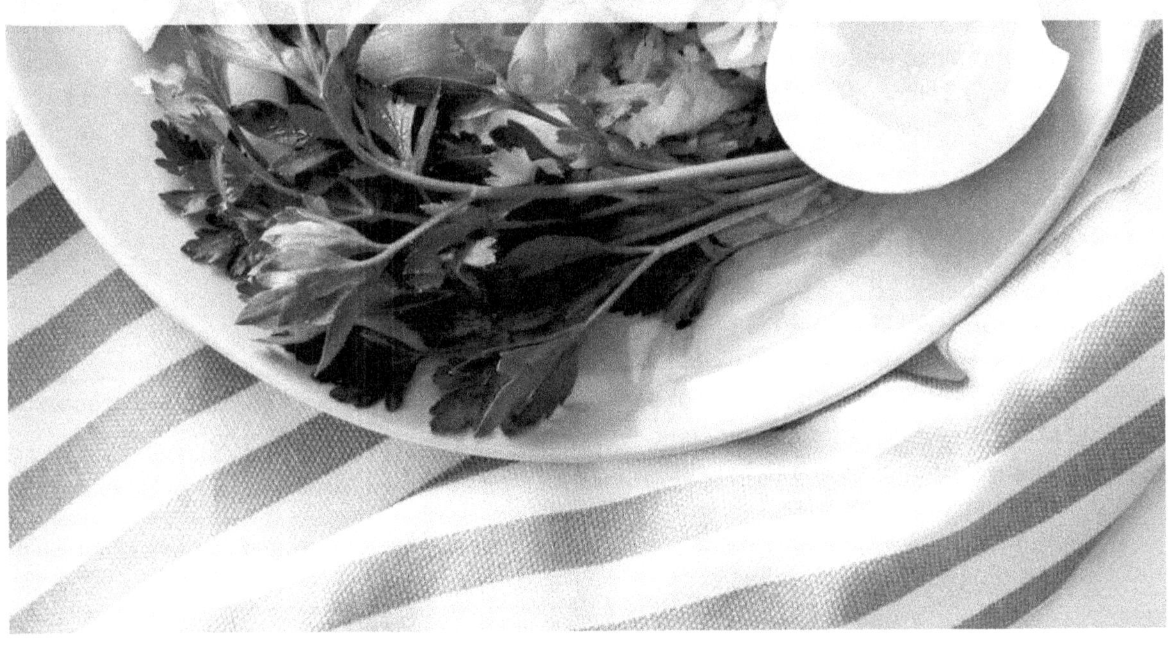
PART TWO:
THE MEAL PLAN

Chapter Four

The Four-Week Meal Plan

Managing diabetes can be daunting, but with this structured four-week meal plan, you can take control of your health while enjoying delicious and nutritious meals. Each week, you'll find a balanced variety of meals designed to stabilize your blood sugar levels, keep you energized, and delight your taste buds. With clear shopping lists and prep tips, you'll find meal planning and preparation easier and more enjoyable. Let's start this journey toward better health together!

Why This Meal Plan Works

This meal plan is crafted with your needs in mind. It emphasizes:

- Low Glycemic Foods: Foods that have a low glycemic index help maintain stable blood sugar levels, preventing spikes and crashes.
- High Fiber Content: Fiber slows down the absorption of sugar and helps improve blood sugar levels. It also promotes digestive health.
- Healthy Fats: Incorporating sources of healthy fats, like avocados and nuts, supports heart health and keeps you satisfied.
- Protein-Rich Meals: Protein helps stabilize blood sugar levels and keeps you feeling full longer, reducing cravings for unhealthy snacks.
- Variety and Balance: A wide range of meals ensures you get all the essential nutrients while keeping your diet interesting and flavorful.

How to Use This Meal Plan

Each week includes:

- A Balanced Meal Plan: Detailed menus for breakfast, lunch, dinner, and snacks, ensuring you get a mix of proteins, healthy fats, and fiber-rich vegetables.
- A Shopping List: Specific quantities of each item needed for a family of four, making grocery shopping straightforward and efficient.
- Prep Tips: Practical advice to help you prepare your meals ahead of time, saving you time and effort during the week.
- Inspiration and Encouragement: Motivational tips to keep you focused and positive about your journey towards better health.

Preparing for Success

To get the most out of this meal plan, here are a few tips:

1. **Plan Your Grocery Shopping:** Use the provided shopping lists to ensure you have all the ingredients you need for the week. This will help you avoid last-minute trips to the store and keep you on track with your meals.
2. **Prep Ahead:** Set aside some time each week to prepare ingredients and meals. This might include chopping vegetables, cooking grains, or marinating proteins. Prepping in advance can make mealtime quicker and less stressful.
3. **Stay Hydrated:** Drink plenty of water throughout the day to stay hydrated and support your overall health.
4. **Listen to Your Body:** Pay attention to how different foods affect your blood sugar levels and adjust your meals as needed. Everyone's body is different, and what works for one person may not work for another.
5. **Stay Positive:** Changing your eating habits can be challenging, but remember that you are making positive changes for your health. Celebrate your progress and stay motivated by focusing on the benefits of a healthier lifestyle.

Let's Get Started!

Embarking on this meal plan is a significant step towards managing your diabetes and improving your overall health. With each meal, you are nourishing your body and making strides towards a healthier future. Enjoy the delicious recipes, embrace the variety of flavors, and take pride in your commitment to your well-being. Let's start this journey towards better health together, one meal at a time!

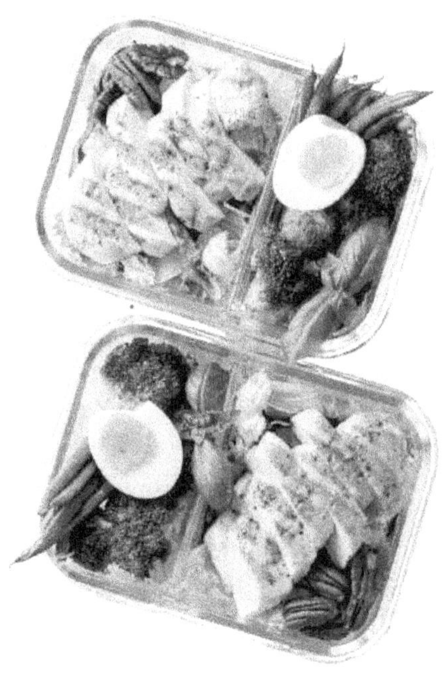

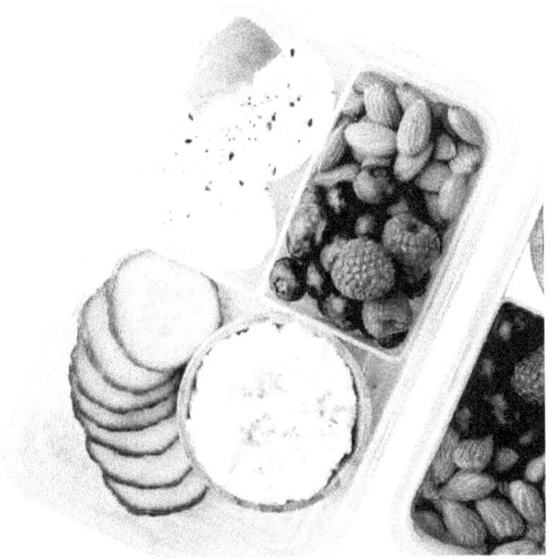

WEEK 1: ESTABLISHING HEALTHY HABITS

This week focuses on creating a solid foundation for your new dietary habits. We start with simple, balanced meals that are rich in nutrients and easy to prepare. The goal is to introduce you to a variety of flavors and textures while keeping your blood sugar levels stable. By establishing healthy habits from the beginning, you'll find it easier to stick to your new lifestyle and enjoy the benefits of improved health and well-being.

This week is all about setting the stage for your journey towards better health. We'll focus on a balanced mix of proteins, healthy fats, and fiber-rich vegetables to create a solid foundation. The meals are simple yet flavorful, ensuring you start on the right foot without feeling overwhelmed. Embrace these changes with an open mind and remember that every small step counts. Enjoy the variety of flavors and the satisfaction of nourishing your body with wholesome foods.

Prep Tips for Week 1:

Sunday Meal Prep:
1. Pre-cook Quinoa and Lentils: Cook a batch of quinoa and lentils to use in various meals throughout the week. This will save you time and make meal preparation quicker.
2. Chop Vegetables: Chop a variety of vegetables for salads, stir-fries, and snacks. Store them in airtight containers in the fridge for easy access.
3. Marinate Meats: Marinate chicken and tofu ahead of time. This not only infuses them with flavor but also makes cooking quicker and easier.
4. Prepare Snacks: Prepare healthy snacks like deviled eggs and spiced nuts. These are perfect for when you need a quick, nutritious bite between meals.
5. Make Breakfasts Ahead: Prepare chia seed pudding and Greek yogurt parfaits the night before. These make for easy and nutritious breakfasts that you can grab and go.

Starting your new meal plan is the first step towards a healthier you. Embrace these changes with an open mind and remember that every small step counts. The journey may seem challenging at first, but each nutritious meal you prepare and enjoy is a victory for your health. By nourishing your body with wholesome foods, you are investing in your well-being and setting yourself up for long-term success. Enjoy the process, celebrate your progress, and look forward to the positive changes ahead. You've got this!

WEEK 1: DIABETIC MEAL PLAN

	BREAKFAST	LUNCH	DINNER	SNACKS
MON	Spinach and Feta Scramble	Spinach and Feta Stuffed Peppers	Baked Salmon with Avocado Salsa	Apple and Walnut Salad
TUES	Greek Yogurt with Nuts and Seeds	Baked Salmon with Asparagus	Grilled Chicken with Quinoa and Spinach	Avocado Deviled Eggs
WED	Veggie-Stuffed Omelet	Chickpea and Vegetable Stir-Fry	Beef and Vegetable Skewers	Cucumber and Hummus Bites
THURS	Chia Seed Pudding with Nuts	Grilled Chicken and Avocado Salad	Turkey Meatballs with Zucchini Noodles	Greek Yogurt and Veggie Dip
FRI	Mushroom and Spinach Breakfast Wrap	Turkey and Avocado Wrap	Chicken and Vegetable Curry	Turkey and Cheese Roll-Ups
SAT	Smoked Salmon and Avocado Toast	Quinoa and Black Bean Salad	Tofu and Vegetable Stir-Fry	Spiced Nuts
SUN	Cottage Cheese and Veggie Bowl	Lentil and Vegetable Soup	Baked Chicken with Brussels Sprouts	Caprese Skewers

GROCERY SHOPPING LIST FOR WEEK 1 DIABETIC MEAL PLAN

MEAT & SEAFOOD

Eggs (3 dozen), Greek yogurt (32 oz), Cottage cheese (16 oz), Feta cheese (8 oz),

Tofu (16 oz), Smoked salmon (16 oz), Salmon fillets (8), Chicken breasts (8)

Ground turkey (2 lbs), Turkey breast (1 lb), Shrimp (2 lbs), Lean beef (1 lb)

GRAINS & LEGUMES

Quinoa (4 cups), Black beans (2 cans)

Lentils (2 cups),

Chia seeds (8 oz)

VEGETABLES

Spinach (14 cups), Mushrooms (8 oz), Avocado (10), Zucchini (6)

Bell peppers (6), Asparagus (4 bunches), Broccoli (2 heads), Brussels sprouts (4 cups)

Tomatoes (6), Cucumbers (4), Carrots (4), Celery (1 bunch)

FRUITS

Apples (8), Oranges (4)

Berries (8 cups),

Lemons (4), Limes (4),

NUTS AND SEEDS

Mixed nuts (16 oz),

Seeds (sunflower,

Chia, flax - 8 oz each)

DAIRY

Greek yogurt (32 oz)

Feta cheese (8 oz)

Cottage cheese (16 oz)

CONDIMENTS & SPICES

Olive oil (16 oz), Cumin

Garlic (2 heads), Salt

Paprika, pepper

WEEK 2: EXPLORING VARIETY

Welcome to Week 2 of your four-week meal plan! This week is all about exploring a variety of meals to keep things interesting and enjoyable. By incorporating different proteins and vegetables, you'll ensure a broad spectrum of nutrients to support your health goals. Variety not only keeps your taste buds excited but also provides a wider range of vitamins, minerals, and other essential nutrients that contribute to overall well-being.

As you move into the second week, you'll begin to see how diverse and enjoyable a balanced diet can be. This week focuses on introducing new flavors and ingredients, ensuring that your meals remain exciting and delicious. Embrace the variety and look forward to discovering new favorites while continuing to stabilize your blood sugar levels and boost your energy.

Prep Tips for Week 2:

1. **Batch-Cook Soups and Stews:**
   - Prepare large batches of soups and stews over the weekend. Store them in portion-sized containers in the fridge or freezer for easy reheating during the week. This will save you time and effort on busy days.
2. **Prepare Breakfast Bowls and Sandwiches the Night Before:**
   - Assemble breakfast bowls and sandwiches the night before to streamline your mornings. This ensures you have a nutritious start to your day without the morning rush.
3. **Keep Pre-Chopped Veggies and Cooked Grains in the Fridge:**
   - Keep a variety of pre-chopped vegetables and cooked grains, such as quinoa and brown rice, in the fridge. This makes it easy to throw together quick salads, stir-fries, and other meals without the hassle of lengthy preparation.

Congratulations on completing Week 1! By now, you should start feeling the positive effects of your new eating habits. This week, we encourage you to embrace the variety of meals and ingredients introduced. Variety is not just the spice of life; it's also a key component of a healthy diet. Trying new foods and recipes can make your meal plan more enjoyable and sustainable in the long run. Remember, each meal you prepare is a step towards better health and well-being.

Embrace the variety of meals in Week 2 and enjoy the new flavors and combinations. Each recipe is designed to support your health goals while keeping your meals exciting and satisfying. Keep exploring, keep preparing, and keep moving towards a healthier you.

Keep up the great work and enjoy the journey!

WEEK 2: DIABETIC MEAL PLAN

	BREAKFAST	LUNCH	DINNER	SNACKS
MON	Avocado and Egg Toast	Tuna and Avocado Salad	Baked Cod with Lemon and Asparagus	Baked Pears with Cinnamon
TUES	Greek Yogurt with Nuts and Seeds	Chickpea and Spinach Curry	Shrimp and Vegetable Stir-Fry	Greek Yogurt Parfait
WED	Tofu Scramble with Veggies	Turkey and Vegetable Lettuce Wraps	Turkey Meatballs with Zucchini Noodles	Berry and Spinach Smoothie
THURS	Smoked Salmon and Avocado Plate	Cauliflower Rice and Shrimp Stir-Fry	Chicken and Vegetable Curry	Pumpkin Protein Bars
FRI	Veggie-Stuffed Omelet	Chicken and Broccoli Stir-Fry	Tofu and Vegetable Stir-Fry	Avocado Deviled Eggs
SAT	Cottage Cheese and Veggie Bowl	Quinoa and Black Bean Salad	Baked Chicken with Brussels Sprouts	Cucumber and Hummus Bites
SUN	Zucchini Fritters	Tofu and Vegetable Stir-Fry	Lentil and Vegetable Stew	Spiced Nuts

GROCERY SHOPPING LIST FOR WEEK 2 DIABETIC MEAL PLAN

PROTEINS

Eggs (3 dozen),
Greek yogurt (32 oz),
Cottage cheese (16 oz),
Feta cheese (8 oz),

Tofu (16 oz),
Smoked salmon (16 oz),
Salmon fillets (8),
Chicken breasts (8),

Ground turkey (2 lbs),
Turkey breast (1 lb),
Shrimp (2 lbs),
Lean beef (1 lb)

GRAINS & LEGUMES

Quinoa (4 cups), Black beans (2 cans)

Lentils (2 cups),

Chia seeds (8 oz)

VEGETABLES

Spinach (14 cups),
Mushrooms (8 oz),
Avocado (10),
Zucchini (6),

Bell peppers (6),
Asparagus (4 bunches),
Broccoli (2 heads),
Brussels sprouts (4 cups),

Tomatoes (6),
Cucumbers (4),
Carrots (4),
Celery (1 bunch)

FRUITS

Apples (8), Oranges (4)

Berries (8 cups),

Lemons (4), Limes (4),

NUTS AND SEEDS

Mixed nuts (16 oz),

Seeds (sunflower, chia, flax - 8 oz each)

DAIRY

Greek yogurt (32 oz)

Feta cheese (8 oz)

Cottage cheese (16 oz)

CONDIMENTS & SPICES

Olive oil (16 oz), Cumin

Garlic (2 heads), Salt

Paprika, pepper

WEEK 3: ENHANCING NUTRITION

You're halfway through your four-week journey! This week is an exciting step towards enhancing your nutrition and overall health. Superfoods are nature's powerhouses, packed with essential nutrients that can help you feel your best. By embracing these foods, you're not just managing your diabetes—you're also giving your body the tools it needs to thrive. Enjoy experimenting with new ingredients and flavors, and remember that each nutrient-packed meal is a step towards better health.

In Week 3, we focus on incorporating superfoods and nutrient-dense ingredients to further enhance your meals. These foods will provide you with the energy and nutrients needed to support your overall health. By introducing a variety of vitamins, minerals, and antioxidants, this week's meal plan aims to boost your immune system, improve digestion, and keep your blood sugar levels stable. Get ready to feel more energized and nourished as you discover the powerful benefits of superfoods.

Prep Tips for Week 3:

1. Batch-Prep Superfood Ingredients:
   - Pre-wash and chop superfoods like kale, spinach, and berries for easy access.
   - Prepare chia seed pudding, overnight oats, and smoothies with superfoods for quick breakfasts and snacks.
2. Make Use of Nutritious Leftovers:
   - Utilize leftovers from nutrient-dense meals to create new dishes. For example, use leftover quinoa in salads or stir-fries.
3. Plan for Variety:
   - Incorporate a range of colors and types of superfoods to ensure a broad spectrum of nutrients. Aim for a colorful plate at each meal.

WEEK 3: DIABETIC MEAL PLAN

	BREAKFAST	LUNCH	DINNER	SNACKS
MON	Almond Flour Pancakes with Greek Yogurt	Grilled Chicken and Avocado Salad	Beef and Vegetable Skewers	Greek Yogurt and Veggie Dip
TUES	Spinach and Feta Scramble	Quinoa and Black Bean Salad	Turkey Meatballs with Zucchini Noodles	Turkey and Cheese Roll-Ups
WED	Avocado and Egg Toast	Turkey and Spinach Wrap	Chicken and Vegetable Curry	Caprese Skewers
THURS	Greek Yogurt with Nuts and Seeds	Lentil and Vegetable Soup	Tofu and Vegetable Stir-Fry	Spinach & Feta Stuffed Mushrooms
FRI	Tofu Scramble with Veggies	Chickpea and Spinach Curry	Baked Chicken with Brussels Sprouts	Edamame with Sea Salt
SAT	Smoked Salmon and Avocado Plate	Turkey and Vegetable Lettuce Wraps	Lentil and Vegetable Stew	Spiced Nuts
SUN	Veggie-Stuffed Omelet	Cauliflower Rice and Shrimp Stir-Fry	Stuffed Bell Peppers with Ground Turkey	Guacamole with Bell Pepper Slices

GROCERY SHOPPING LIST FOR WEEK 3 DIABETIC MEAL PLAN

PROTEINS

Eggs (3 dozen),
Greek yogurt (32 oz),
Cottage cheese (16 oz),
Feta cheese (8 oz),

Tofu (16 oz),
Smoked salmon (16 oz),
Salmon fillets (8),
Chicken breasts (8),

Ground turkey (2 lbs),
Turkey breast (1 lb),
Shrimp (2 lbs),
Lean beef (1 lb)

GRAINS & LEGUMES

Quinoa (4 cups), Black beans (2 cans)   Lentils (2 cups),   Chia seeds (8 oz)

VEGETABLES

Spinach (14 cups),
Mushrooms (8 oz),
Avocado (10),
Zucchini (6),

Bell peppers (6),
Asparagus (4 bunches),
Broccoli (2 heads),
Brussels sprouts (4 cups),

Tomatoes (6),
Cucumbers (4),
Carrots (4),
Celery (1 bunch)

FRUITS

Apples (8), Oranges (4)   Berries (8 cups),   Lemons (4), Limes (4),

NUTS AND SEEDS

Mixed nuts (16 oz),   Seeds (sunflower, chia, flax - 8 oz each)

DAIRY

Greek yogurt (32 oz)   Feta cheese (8 oz)   Cottage cheese (16 oz)

CONDIMENTS & SPICES

Olive oil (16 oz), Cumin   Garlic (2 heads), Salt   Paprika, pepper

WEEK 4: MASTERING YOUR NEW LIFESTYLE

You're in the final stretch of your four-week journey! This week is about mastering your new lifestyle and solidifying the healthy habits you've developed. You've learned how to manage your diabetes with balanced, nutritious meals, and now it's time to refine those skills and ensure they become a natural part of your routine.

In Week 4, we focus on variety and balance, ensuring your meals continue to provide the nutrients you need to thrive. This week's plan includes a mix of your favorite recipes from the previous weeks, along with some new options to keep things interesting. The goal is to reinforce your newfound habits and make healthy eating second nature.

Prep Tips for Week 4:

1. Finalize Your Routine:
   - Identify the recipes you enjoyed most and plan to incorporate them regularly.
   - Create a flexible meal plan that allows for variety while maintaining balance.
2. Optimize Your Prep:
   - Continue to batch-cook ingredients like grains, proteins, and veggies for easy meal assembly.
   - Prepare grab-and-go snacks to keep your energy levels stable throughout the day.
3. Embrace Balance:
   - Focus on balanced meals with a mix of proteins, healthy fats, and fiber-rich vegetables.
   - Adjust portions and ingredients to fit your personal preferences and nutritional needs.

Congratulations on making it to Week 4! You've come a long way in your journey toward better health. By now, you've experienced the benefits of a balanced diet in managing your diabetes and improving your overall well-being. Keep up the great work, stay committed to your new habits, and enjoy the positive changes you've made.

Remember, every healthy choice you make is a step toward a healthier, happier life.

WEEK 4: DIABETIC MEAL PLAN

	BREAKFAST	LUNCH	DINNER	SNACKS
MON	Egg and Avocado Breakfast Bowl	Chicken and Broccoli Stir-Fry	Grilled Shrimp Tacos with Avocado	Apple and Walnut Salad
TUES	Smoked Salmon and Avocado Toast	Quinoa and Black Bean Salad	Eggplant Parmesan	Avocado Deviled Eggs
WED	Egg and Veggie Breakfast Muffins	Grilled Chicken and Avocado Salad	Turkey and Spinach Stuffed Portobello Mushrooms	Cucumber and Hummus Bites
THURS	Almond Flour Pancakes with Greek Yogurt	Turkey and Spinach Wrap	Lemon Herb Grilled Chicken	Greek Yogurt and Veggie Dip
FRI	Spinach and Feta Scramble	Lentil and Vegetable Soup	Spaghetti Squash with Tomato and Basil	Spiced Nuts
SAT	Avocado and Egg Toast	Tuna and Avocado Salad	Salmon with Asparagus and Lemon	Lentil and Veggie Lettuce Wraps
SUN	Greek Yogurt with Nuts and Seeds	Tofu and Vegetable Stir-Fry	Chicken and Broccoli Stir-Fry	Guacamole with Bell Pepper Slices

GROCERY SHOPPING LIST FOR WEEK 4 DIABETIC MEAL PLAN

PROTEINS

Eggs (3 dozen), Greek yogurt (32 oz), Cottage cheese (16 oz), Feta cheese (8 oz),

Tofu (16 oz), Smoked salmon (16 oz), Salmon fillets (8), Chicken breasts (8),

Ground turkey (2 lbs), Turkey breast (1 lb), Shrimp (2 lbs), Lean beef (1 lb)

GRAINS & LEGUMES

Quinoa (4 cups), Black beans (2 cans)

Lentils (2 cups),

Chia seeds (8 oz)

VEGETABLES

Spinach (14 cups), Mushrooms (8 oz), Avocado (10), Zucchini (6),

Bell peppers (6), Asparagus (4 bunches), Broccoli (2 heads), Brussels sprouts (4 cups),

Tomatoes (6), Cucumbers (4), Carrots (4), Celery (1 bunch)

FRUITS

Apples (8), Oranges (4)

Berries (8 cups),

Lemons (4), Limes (4),

NUTS AND SEEDS

Mixed nuts (16 oz),

Seeds (sunflower, chia, flax - 8 oz each)

DAIRY

Greek yogurt (32 oz)

Feta cheese (8 oz)

Cottage cheese (16 oz)

CONDIMENTS & SPICES

Olive oil (16 oz), Cumin

Garlic (2 heads), Salt

Paprika, pepper

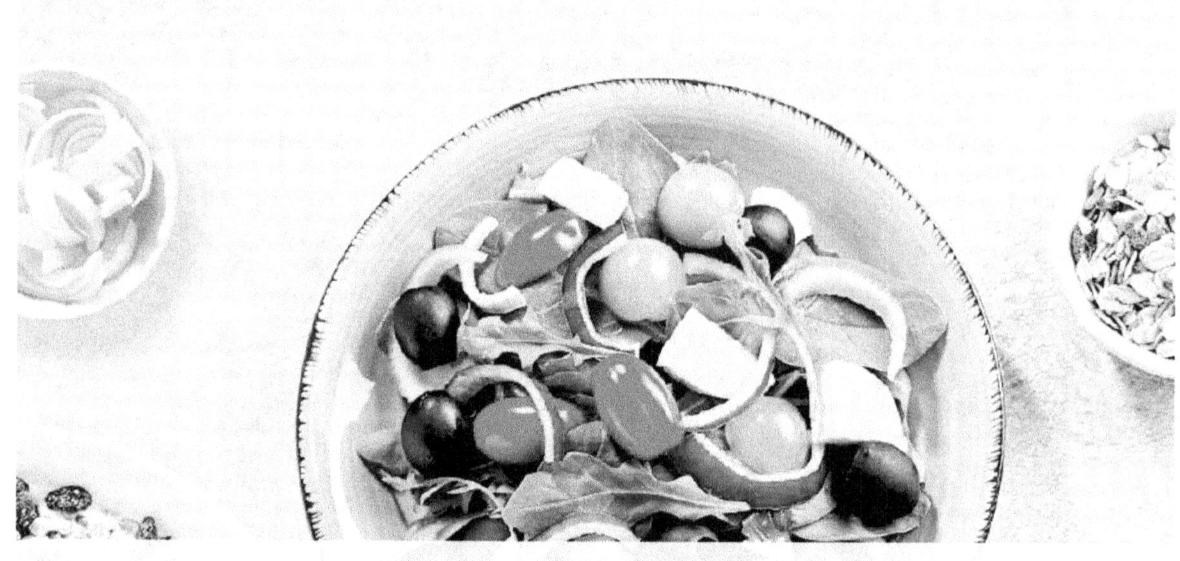

PART THREE:
THE RECIPES

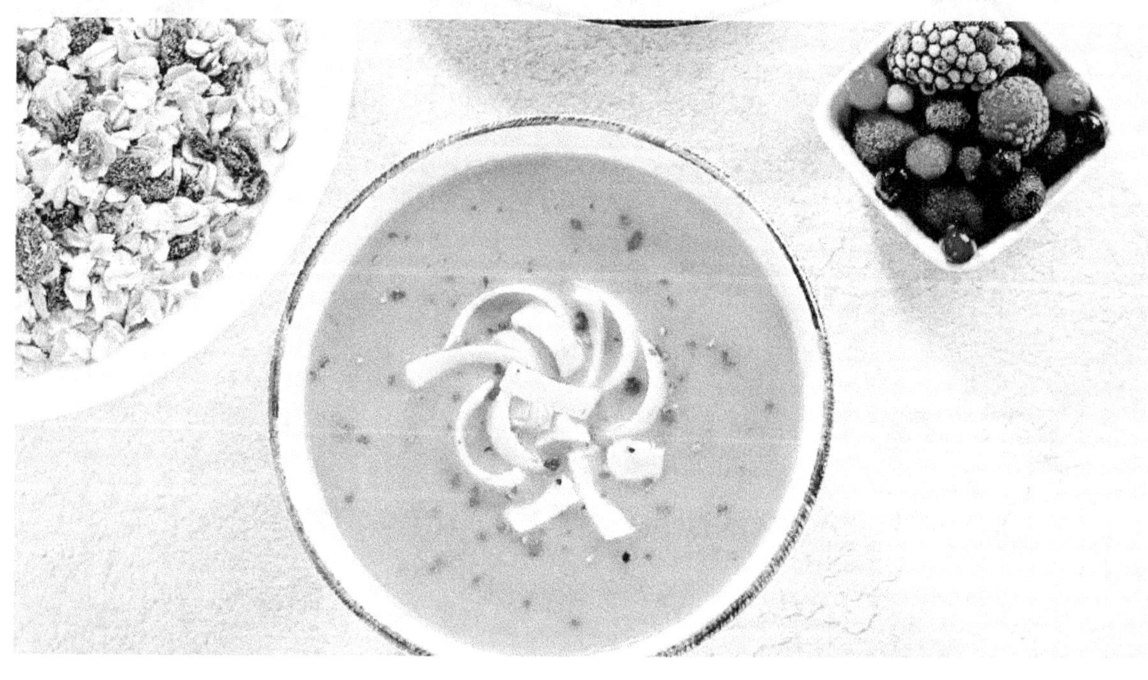

Chapter Five

Breakfast Recipes

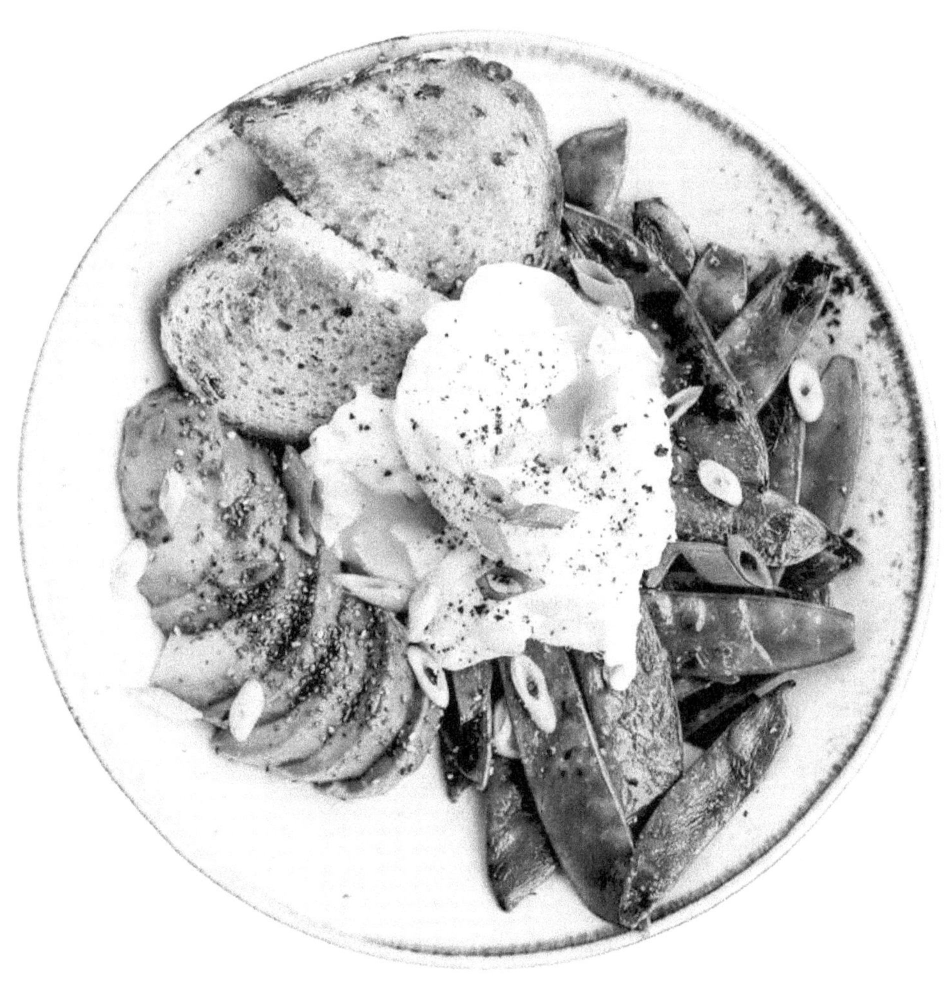

Spinach and Feta Scramble

This quick and easy spinach and feta scramble is a perfect start to your day, offering a protein-packed, savory breakfast that will keep you energized and your blood sugar steady.

Servings: 1 | Prep Time: 5 mins | Cook Time: 5 mins | Carbs per Serving: 3g

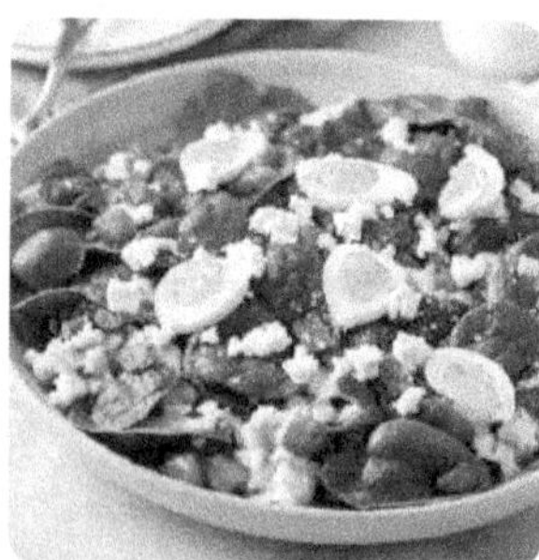

Ingredients

- 2 large eggs
- 1 cup fresh spinach, chopped
- 1/4 cup feta cheese, crumbled
- 1 tbsp olive oil
- Salt and pepper to taste

Directions

1. Heat the olive oil in a skillet over medium heat.
2. Add the chopped spinach and sauté until wilted.
3. Beat the eggs in a bowl and pour them into the skillet.
4. Cook the eggs, stirring gently, until they are set but still soft.
5. Add the feta cheese and stir to combine.
6. Season with salt and pepper to taste and serve hot.

Ingredient Tips:

- Spinach: Low in carbohydrates and high in fiber, spinach has a low glycemic index, helping to manage blood sugar levels.
- Feta Cheese: Provides protein and healthy fats, but use in moderation due to its sodium content.

Avocado and Egg Toast

A simple yet delicious breakfast option that combines the creaminess of avocado with the protein of eggs on whole grain toast.

Servings: 1 | Prep Time: 5 mins | Cook Time: 5 mins | Carbs per Serving: 18g

Ingredients

- 1 slice whole grain bread
- 1/2 avocado, mashed
- 1 large egg
- 1 tbsp olive oil
- Salt and pepper to taste

Directions

1. Toast the whole grain bread.
2. Heat olive oil in a skillet over medium heat and fry the egg to your desired doneness.
3. Spread the mashed avocado on the toasted bread.
4. Top with the fried egg.
5. Season with salt and pepper to taste and serve immediately.

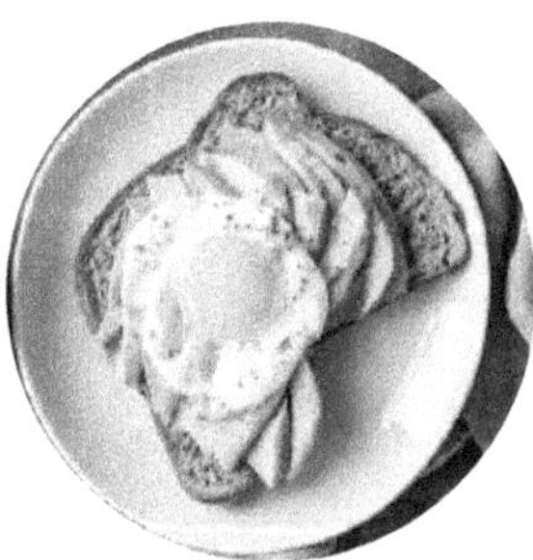

Ingredient Tips:

- Avocado: Rich in healthy fats and fiber, avocado helps increase satiety and manage blood sugar levels.
- Whole Grain Bread: Provides complex carbohydrates with a lower glycemic index compared to refined grains, helping to maintain steady blood sugar levels.

Greek Yogurt with Nuts and Seeds

This creamy Greek yogurt breakfast is topped with a mix of nuts and seeds, providing a delicious, protein-packed start to your day.

Servings: 1 | Prep Time: 5 mins | Cook Time: 0 mins | Carbs per Serving: 1 15g

INGREDIENTS

- 1 cup full-fat Greek yogurt
- 1 tbsp chia seeds
- 1 tbsp flaxseeds
- 2 tbsp chopped almonds

DIRECTIONS

1. Place the Greek yogurt in a bowl.
2. Top with chia seeds, flaxseeds, chopped almonds, and walnuts.
3. Add fresh berries if desired.
4. Mix gently and enjoy.

Ingredient Tips:

- Greek Yogurt: High in protein and lower in carbohydrates than regular yogurt, making it a great choice for blood sugar management.
- Nuts and Seeds: Provide healthy fats and fiber, which help to slow the absorption of sugar into the bloodstream.

Tofu Scramble with Veggies

A vegan-friendly tofu scramble that's packed with protein and fiber-rich vegetables, perfect for a healthy and balanced breakfast.

Servings: 2 | Prep Time: 10 mins | Cook Time: 10 mins | Carbs per Serving: 8g

Ingredients

- 1 block firm tofu, crumbled
- 1 cup mixed bell peppers, diced
- 1/2 cup red onion, diced
- 1 cup spinach, chopped
- 1 tbsp olive oil

Directions

1. Heat the olive oil in a skillet over medium heat.
2. Add the red onion and bell peppers and sauté until soft.
3. Add the crumbled tofu and turmeric, stirring to combine.
4. Cook for about 5 minutes, stirring occasionally.
5. Add the chopped spinach and cook until wilted.
6. Season with salt and pepper to taste and serve hot.

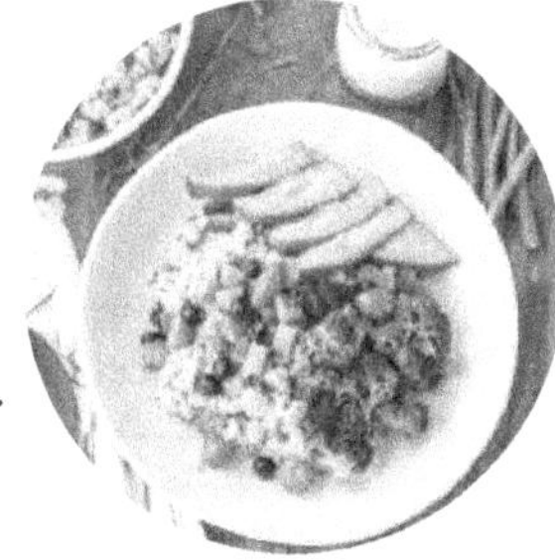

Ingredient Tips:

- Tofu: A great source of plant-based protein and has a low glycemic index, making it ideal for blood sugar control.
- Turmeric: Contains curcumin, which has anti-inflammatory properties and can help manage blood sugar levels.

Smoked Salmon and Avocado Plate

This elegant breakfast plate features smoked salmon and avocado, offering a savory combination that's rich in protein and healthy fats.

Servings: 1 | Prep Time: 5 mins | Cook Time: 0 mins | Carbs per Serving: 6g

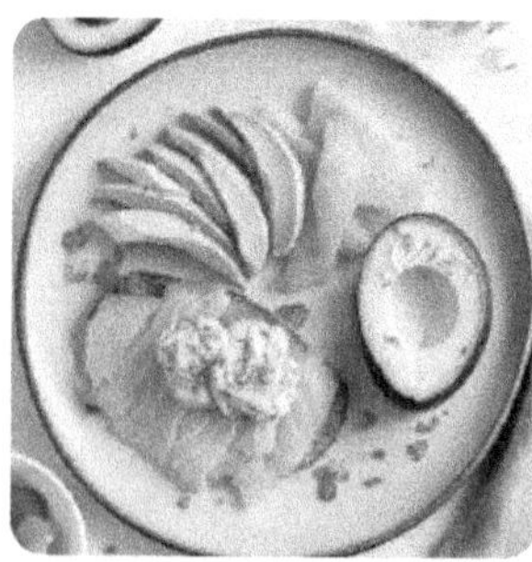

Ingredients

- 3 oz smoked salmon
- 1/2 avocado, sliced
- 1 tbsp capers
- 1 tbsp red onion, thinly sliced
- 1 tbsp lemon juice
- Salt and pepper to taste

Directions

1. Arrange the smoked salmon and avocado slices on a plate.
2. Sprinkle with capers and red onion.
3. Drizzle with lemon juice.
4. Season with salt and pepper to taste and serve.

Ingredient Tips:

- Smoked Salmon: High in protein and omega-3 fatty acids, which help to reduce inflammation and improve heart health.
- Avocado: Provides healthy fats and fiber, aiding in satiety and blood sugar management.

Veggie-Stuffed Omelet

A hearty omelet packed with fiber-rich vegetables and cheese for a satisfying and balanced breakfast.

Servings: 1 | Prep Time: 5 mins | Cook Time: 10 mins | Carbs per Serving: 6g

Ingredients

- 2 large eggs
- 1/4 cup diced bell peppers
- 1/4 cup diced tomatoes
- 1/4 cup chopped spinach
- 1/4 cup shredded cheese (cheddar or mozzarella)
- 1 tbsp olive oil
- Salt and pepper to taste

Directions

1. Beat the eggs in a bowl and set aside.
2. Heat the olive oil in a skillet over medium heat.
3. Add the bell peppers, tomatoes, and spinach, and sauté until soft.
4. Pour the beaten eggs into the skillet and let them cook until they begin to set.
5. Sprinkle the shredded cheese over the eggs.
6. Fold the omelet in half and cook until the cheese is melted.
7. Season with salt and pepper to taste and serve hot.

Ingredient Tips:

- Eggs: An excellent source of protein and nutrients that help keep you full and satisfied.
- Vegetables: Low in carbohydrates and high in fiber, they help to maintain steady blood sugar levels.

Cottage Cheese and Veggie Bowl

A refreshing and nutritious bowl of cottage cheese paired with a variety of fresh vegetables for a protein-rich breakfast.

Servings: 1 | Prep Time: 5 mins | Cook Time: 0 mins | Carbs per Serving: 8g

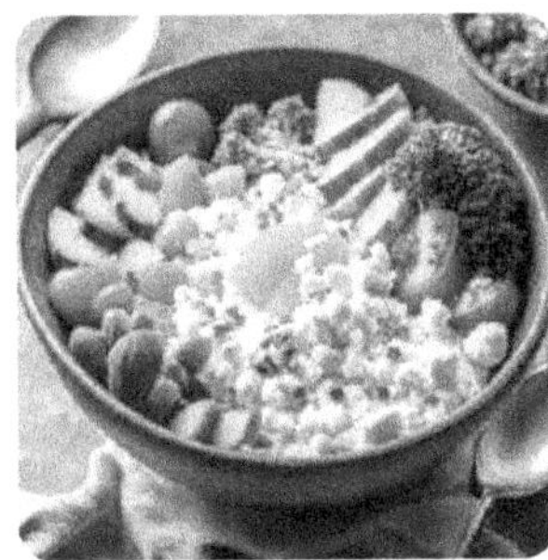

Ingredients

- 1 cup cottage cheese
- 1/2 cup cherry tomatoes, halved
- 1/2 cucumber, sliced
- 1/4 cup chopped bell peppers
- 1 tbsp olive oil
- Salt and pepper to taste

Directions

1. Place the cottage cheese in a bowl.
2. Top with cherry tomatoes, cucumber, and bell peppers.
3. Drizzle with olive oil.
4. Season with salt and pepper to taste and serve

Ingredient Tips:

- Cottage Cheese: High in protein and low in carbohydrates, making it an excellent option for blood sugar management.
- Vegetables: Adding a variety of fresh vegetables increases the fiber content, helping to slow the absorption of sugars.

Mushroom and Spinach Breakfast Wrap

A tasty and nutritious wrap filled with sautéed mushrooms, spinach, and scrambled eggs for a balanced breakfast.

Servings: 1 | Prep Time: 5 mins | Cook Time: 10 mins | Carbs per Serving: 2g

Ingredients

- 2 large eggs
- 1 cup mushrooms, sliced
- 1 cup spinach, chopped
- 1 tbsp olive oil
- 1 whole grain tortilla
- Salt and pepper to taste

Directions

1. Heat the olive oil in a skillet over medium heat.
2. Add the mushrooms and sauté until they are soft and browned.
3. Add the spinach and cook until wilted.
4. Beat the eggs in a bowl and pour them into the skillet.
5. Cook the eggs, stirring gently, until they are set but still soft.
6. Warm the tortilla in a separate pan or microwave.
7. Fill the tortilla with the egg mixture and wrap it up.
8. Season with salt and pepper to taste and serve.

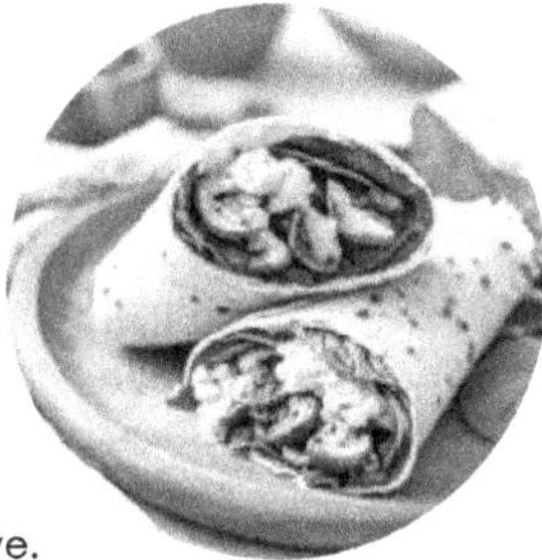

Ingredient Tips:

- Whole Grain Tortilla: Provides complex carbohydrates with a lower glycemic index compared to refined grains.
- Mushrooms: Low in calories and carbohydrates, they add a savory flavor and nutrients to your meal.

Zucchini Fritters

These savory zucchini fritters are a delicious and healthy breakfast option, packed with vegetables and protein.

Servings: 1 | Prep Time: 5 mins | Cook Time: 0 mins | Carbs per Serving: 8g

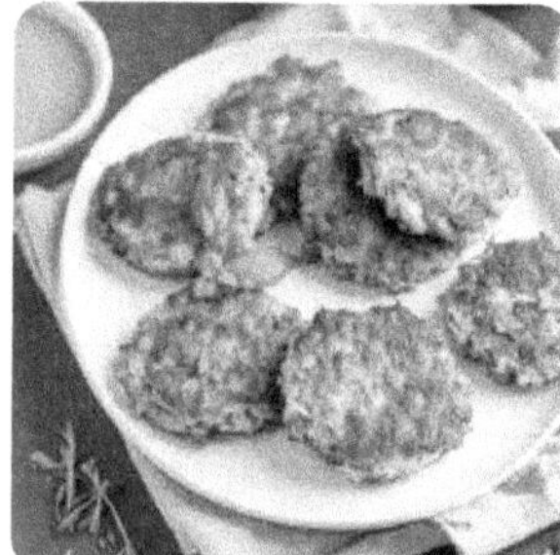

Ingredients

- 2 cups grated zucchini
- 2 large eggs
- 1/4 cup almond flour
- 1/4 cup grated Parmesan cheese
- 1 tbsp olive oil
- Salt and pepper to taste

Directions

1. Squeeze the excess moisture from the grated zucchini.
2. In a bowl, mix the zucchini, eggs, almond flour, Parmesan cheese, salt, and pepper.
3. Heat the olive oil in a skillet over medium heat.
4. Scoop small portions of the mixture into the skillet and flatten them with a spatula.
5. Cook the fritters for about 3-4 minutes on each side or until golden brown.
6. Remove from the skillet and drain on paper towels.
7. Serve hot.

Ingredient Tips:

- Cottage Cheese: High in protein and low in carbohydrates, making it Zucchini: Low in carbohydrates and high in fiber, making it a great choice for managing blood sugar levels.
- Almond Flour: Provides healthy fats and protein, and has a low glycemic index.

Turkey and Avocado Breakfast Sandwich

A hearty and satisfying breakfast sandwich made with lean turkey, avocado, and a whole grain English muffin.

Servings: 1 | Prep Time: 5 mins | Cook Time: 5 mins | Carbs per Serving: 28g

Ingredients

- 1 whole grain English muffin, split and toasted
- 2 oz lean turkey breast
- 1/2 avocado, sliced
- 1 tbsp Greek yogurt
- 1 tbsp Dijon mustard
- Salt and pepper to taste

Directions

1. Toast the whole grain English muffin halves.
2. Spread Greek yogurt and Dijon mustard on one half of the muffin.
3. Layer the turkey breast and avocado slices on top.
4. Season with salt and pepper to taste.
5. Top with the other half of the muffin and serve immediately.

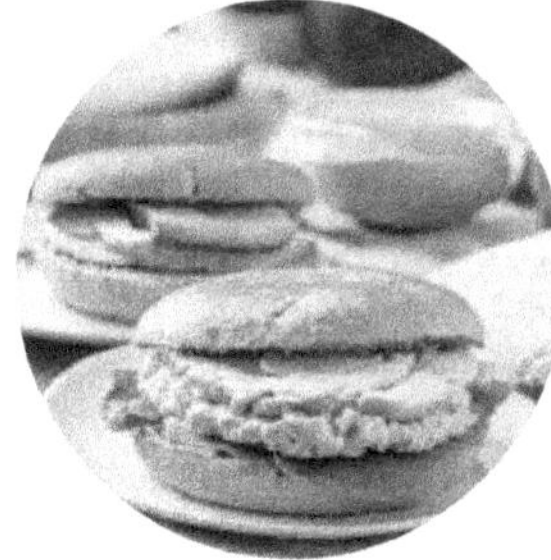

Ingredient Tips:

- Lean Turkey Breast: High in protein and low in fat, making it an excellent option for a balanced breakfast.
- Whole Grain English Muffin: Provides complex carbohydrates and fiber, which help maintain steady blood sugar levels.

Cauliflower Rice and Egg Bowl

A nutritious breakfast bowl made with cauliflower rice, scrambled eggs, and fresh vegetables for a low-carb, high-protein meal.

Servings: 2 | Prep Time: 10 mins | Cook Time: 10 mins | Carbs per Serving: 6g

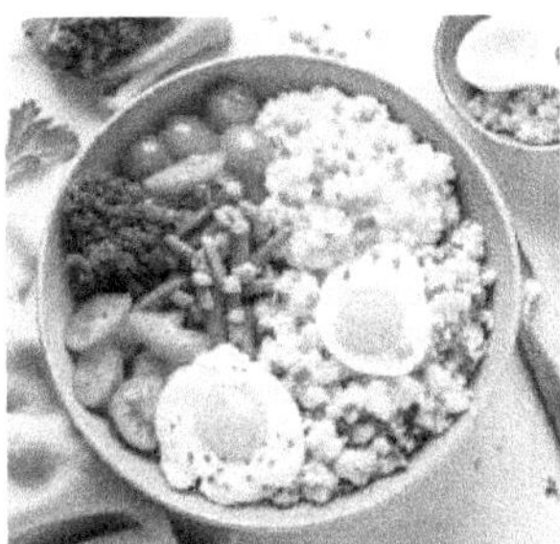

Ingredients

- 2 cups cauliflower rice
- 2 large eggs
- 1/2 cup diced bell peppers
- 1/2 cup diced tomatoes
- 1/4 cup chopped spinach
- 1 tbsp olive oil
- Salt and pepper to taste

Directions

1. Heat the olive oil in a skillet over medium heat.
2. Add the bell peppers and tomatoes and sauté until soft.
3. Add the cauliflower rice and cook until heated through.
4. In a separate pan, scramble the eggs until cooked through.
5. Combine the scrambled eggs with the cauliflower rice and vegetable mixture.
6. Stir in the chopped spinach and cook until wilted.
7. Season with salt and pepper to taste and serve.

Ingredient Tips:

- Cauliflower Rice: Low in carbohydrates and high in fiber, making it a perfect alternative to regular rice for managing blood sugar levels.
- Vegetables: Adding a variety of vegetables increases the fiber content, aiding in digestion and blood sugar control.

Chia Seed Pudding with Nuts

A creamy and nutritious chia seed pudding topped with nuts for a delicious, protein-rich breakfast.

Servings: 2 | Prep Time: 5 mins | Cook Time: 0 mins | Carbs per Serving: 12g

Ingredients

- 1/4 cup chia seeds
- 1 cup unsweetened almond milk
- 1/2 tsp vanilla extract
- 1/4 cup mixed nuts (almonds, walnuts, pecans)
- Fresh berries (optional)
- Salt to taste

Directions

1. In a bowl, mix the chia seeds, almond milk, vanilla extract, and a pinch of salt.
2. Stir well to combine and let sit for about 5 minutes.
3. Stir again to prevent clumping and refrigerate for at least 2 hours or overnight.
4. Top the chia seed pudding with mixed nuts and fresh berries if desired.
5. Serve cold.

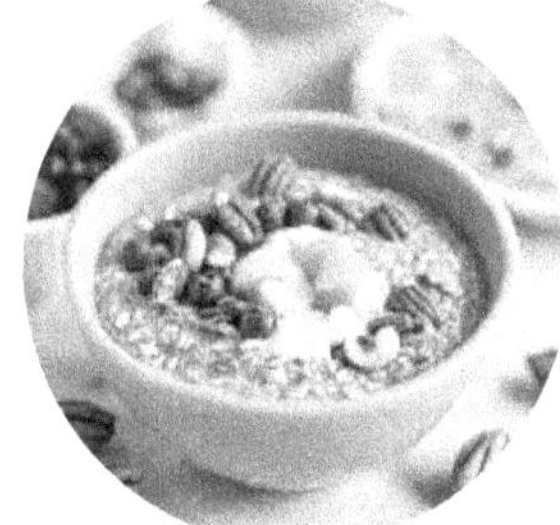

Ingredient Tips:

- Chia Seeds: High in fiber and omega-3 fatty acids, which help to maintain steady blood sugar levels.
- Nuts: Provide healthy fats and protein, helping to keep you full and satisfied.

Avocado & Chickpea Breakfast Salad

<table><tr><td>

A refreshing and protein-packed breakfast salad with avocado, chickpeas, and fresh vegetables.

</td><td>

NUTRIENT CONTENT (PER SERVING):

- Calories: 300
- Total Fat: 16g
- Protein: 8g
- Carbohydrates: 22g
- Sugars: 4g
- Fiber: 10g
- Sodium: 200mg

</td></tr></table>

Servings: 2 | Prep Time: 10 mins | Cook Time: 0 mins | Carbs per Serving: 22g

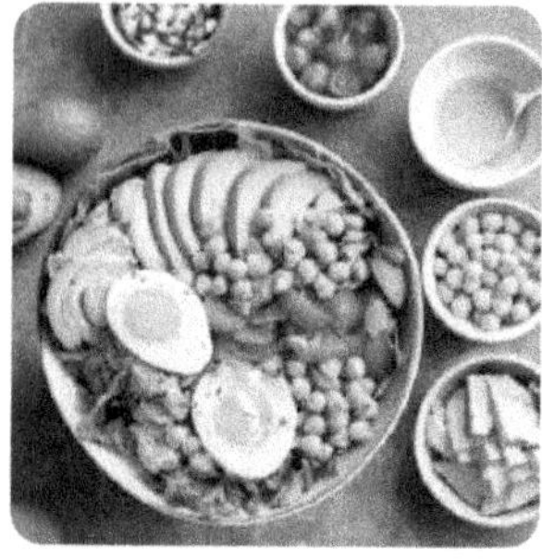

Ingredients

- 1/2 avocado, diced
- 1 cup cooked chickpeas
- 1/2 cup cherry tomatoes, halved
- 1/2 cucumber, sliced
- 1/4 cup red onion, thinly sliced
- 1 tbsp olive oil
- 1 tbsp lemon juice
- Salt and pepper to taste

Directions

1. In a large bowl, combine the diced avocado, chickpeas, cherry tomatoes, cucumber, and red onion.
2. Drizzle with olive oil and lemon juice.
3. Toss gently to combine.
4. Season with salt and pepper to taste and serve immediately.

Ingredient Tips:

- Chickpeas: High in protein and fiber, helping to keep you full and manage blood sugar levels.
- Avocado: Provides healthy fats and fiber, aiding in satiety and blood sugar control

---

Salmon and Spinach Frittata

A delicious and nutritious frittata made with smoked salmon and spinach for a protein-rich breakfast.

NUTRIENT CONTENT (PER SERVING):

- Calories: 200
- Total Fat: 14g
- Protein: 16g
- Carbohydrates: 2g
- Sugars: 1g
- Fiber: 1g
- Sodium: 350mg

Servings: 4 | Prep Time: 10 mins | Cook Time :20 mins | Carbs per Serving: 2g

Ingredients

- 6 large eggs
- 1/2 cup smoked salmon, chopped
- 1 cup spinach, chopped
- 1/4 cup chopped red onion
- 1 tbsp olive oil
- Salt and pepper to taste

Directions

1. Preheat the oven to 375°F (190°C).
2. In a large oven-safe skillet, heat the olive oil over medium heat.
3. Add the chopped red onion and sauté until soft.
4. Add the chopped spinach and cook until wilted.
5. In a bowl, beat the eggs and season with salt and pepper.
6. Pour the beaten eggs into the skillet and stir gently to combine with the vegetables.
7. Sprinkle the chopped smoked salmon on top.
8. Transfer the skillet to the oven and bake for 15-20 minutes, or until the frittata is set and golden brown.
9. Allow to cool slightly before slicing and serving.

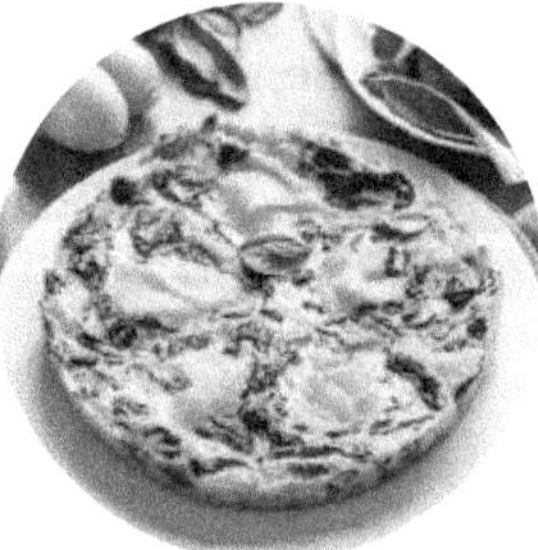

Ingredient Tips:

- Smoked Salmon: High in protein and omega-3 fatty acids, which help to reduce inflammation and improve heart health.
- Spinach: Low in carbohydrates and high in fiber, making it a great choice for managing blood sugar levels.

Quinoa Breakfast Bowl

A wholesome breakfast bowl featuring quinoa, eggs, and fresh vegetables for a balanced and nutritious meal.

Servings: 1 | Prep Time: 10 mins | Cook Time: 10 mins | Carbs per Serving: 26g

<table>
<tr><td></td><td colspan="2">NUTRIENT CONTENT (PER SERVING):</td></tr>
<tr><td></td><td>• Calories: 350
• Total Fat: 20g
• Protein: 14g
• Carbohydrates: 26g</td><td>• Sugars: 3g
• Fiber: 8g
• Sodium: 200mg</td></tr>
</table>

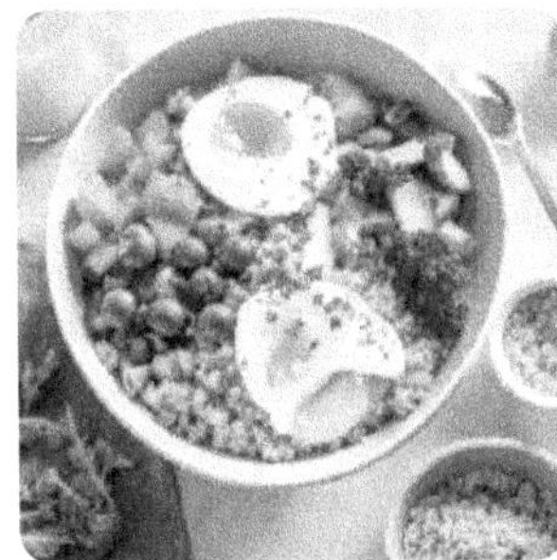

Ingredients

- 1/2 cup cooked quinoa
- 2 large eggs
- 1/2 avocado, sliced
- 1/2 cup cherry tomatoes, halved
- 1/4 cup chopped bell peppers
- 1 tbsp olive oil
- Salt and pepper to taste

Directions

1. Cook the quinoa according to package instructions and set aside.
2. Heat the olive oil in a skillet over medium heat.
3. Add the chopped bell peppers and sauté until soft.
4. In a separate pan, scramble the eggs until cooked through.
5. In a bowl, combine the cooked quinoa, scrambled eggs, bell peppers, cherry tomatoes, and avocado slices.
6. Season with salt and pepper to taste and serve.

Ingredient Tips:

- Quinoa: A whole grain that's high in protein and fiber, helping to maintain steady blood sugar levels.
- Avocado: Provides healthy fats and fiber, aiding in satiety and blood sugar control.

Lentil and Veggie Stir-Fry

A savory breakfast stir-fry made with lentils and fresh vegetables for a protein and fiber-rich start to your day.

Servings: 2 | Prep Time: 10 mins | Cook Time :10 mins | Carbs per Serving: 20g

NUTRIENT CONTENT (PER SERVING):

- Calories: 180
- Total Fat: 8g
- Protein: 10g
- Carbohydrates: 20g
- Sugars: 3g
- Fiber: 8g
- Sodium: 150mg

Ingredients

- 1 cup cooked lentils
- 1/2 cup diced bell peppers
- 1/2 cup diced tomatoes
- 1/4 cup chopped spinach
- 1 tbsp olive oil
- Salt and pepper to taste

Directions

1. Heat the olive oil in a skillet over medium heat.
2. Add the bell peppers and tomatoes and sauté until soft.
3. Add the cooked lentils and stir to combine.
4. Stir in the chopped spinach and cook until wilted.
5. Season with salt and pepper to taste and serve hot.

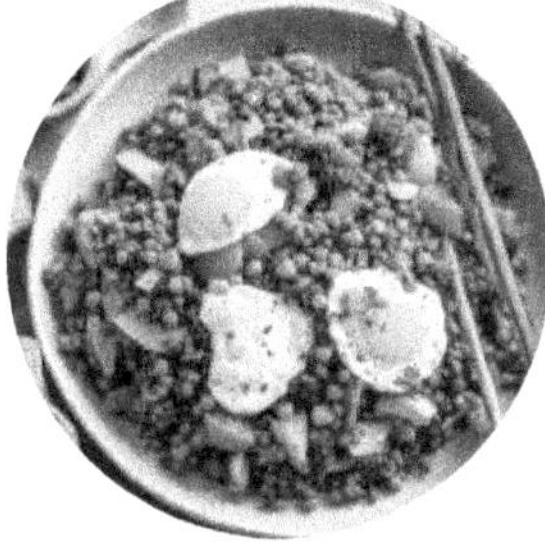

Ingredient Tips:

- Lentils: High in protein and fiber, making them an excellent option for managing blood sugar levels.
- Vegetables: Adding a variety of vegetables increases the fiber content, aiding in digestion and blood sugar control.

Egg and Avocado Breakfast Bowl

A simple and delicious breakfast bowl featuring eggs, avocado, and fresh vegetables for a balanced and nutritious meal.

Servings: 1 | Prep Time: 10 mins | Cook Time: 5 mins | Carbs per Serving: 10g

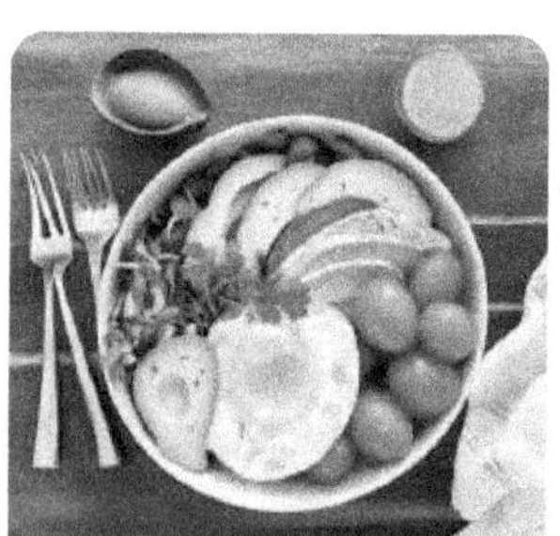

Ingredients

- 2 large eggs
- 1/2 avocado, sliced
- 1/2 cup cherry tomatoes, halved
- 1/4 cup chopped spinach
- 1 tbsp olive oil
- Salt and pepper to taste

Directions

1. Heat the olive oil in a skillet over medium heat.
2. Add the chopped spinach and sauté until wilted.
3. In a separate pan, scramble the eggs until cooked through.
4. In a bowl, combine the scrambled eggs, sautéed spinach, cherry tomatoes, and avocado slices.
5. Season with salt and pepper to taste and serve.

Ingredient Tips:

- Eggs: Provide high-quality protein and essential nutrients that help keep you full and satisfied.
- Avocado: Provides healthy fats and fiber, aiding in satiety and blood sugar control.

Smoked Salmon and Avocado Toast

A delicious and protein-packed breakfast toast topped with smoked salmon and avocado for a nutritious start to your day.

Servings: 1 | Prep Time: 5 mins | Cook Time :5 mins | Carbs per Serving: 20g

Ingredients

- 1 slice whole grain bread
- 1/2 avocado, mashed
- 2 oz smoked salmon
- 1/4 cup sliced cucumber
- 1 tbsp cream cheese (optional)
- Salt and pepper to taste

Directions

1. Toast the whole grain bread slice.
2. Spread the mashed avocado on the toast.
3. Layer the smoked salmon and sliced cucumber on top.
4. Add a dollop of cream cheese if desired.
5. Season with salt and pepper to taste and serve.

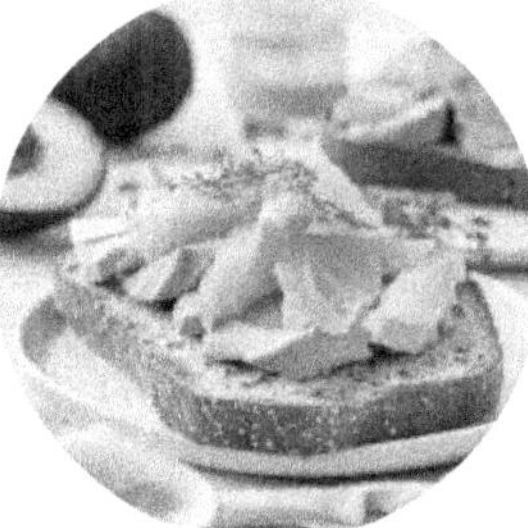

Ingredient Tips:

- Whole Grain Bread: Provides complex carbohydrates and fiber, which help maintain steady blood sugar levels.
- Smoked Salmon: High in protein and omega-3 fatty acids, which help to reduce inflammation and improve heart health.

Egg and Veggie Breakfast Muffins

These egg and veggie breakfast muffins are perfect for meal prep, providing a protein-packed and fiber-rich breakfast option.

Servings: 6 | Prep Time: 10 mins | Cook Time: 25 mins | Carbs per Serving: 2g

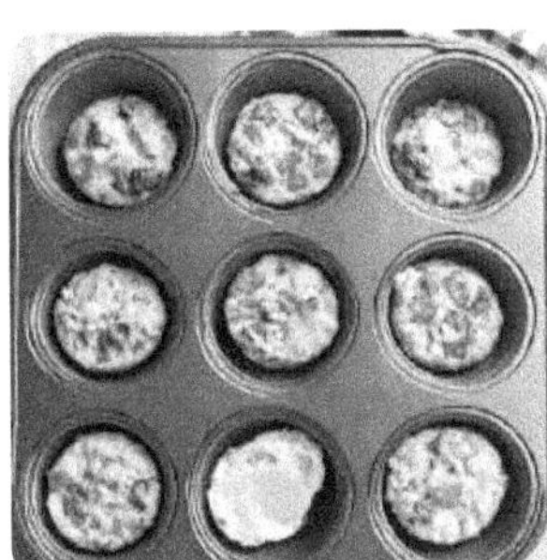

Ingredients

- 6 large eggs
- 1/2 cup diced bell peppers
- 1/2 cup diced tomatoes
- 1/2 cup chopped spinach
- 1/4 cup shredded cheese (optional)
- Salt and pepper to taste
- Non-stick cooking spray

Directions

1. Preheat the oven to 375°F (190°C).
2. Spray a muffin tin with non-stick cooking spray.
3. In a large bowl, beat the eggs and season with salt and pepper.
4. Stir in the bell peppers, tomatoes, and spinach.
5. Pour the egg mixture into the muffin tin, filling each cup about three-quarters full.
6. Sprinkle shredded cheese on top if desired.
7. Bake for 20-25 minutes, or until the eggs are set.
8. Allow to cool slightly before removing from the muffin tin and serving.

Ingredient Tips:

- Eggs: Provide high-quality protein and essential nutrients that help keep you full and satisfied.
- Vegetables: Adding a variety of vegetables increases the fiber content, aiding in digestion and blood sugar control.

Almond Flour Pancakes with Greek Yogurt

Enjoy these low-carb, high-protein almond flour pancakes topped with Greek yogurt for a nutritious and satisfying breakfast.

Servings: 2 | Prep Time: 10 mins | Cook Time: 10 mins | Carbs per Serving: 12g

Ingredients

- 1 cup almond flour
- 2 large eggs
- 1/4 cup unsweetened almond milk
- 1 tsp baking powder
- 1/2 tsp vanilla extract
- 1/2 cup full-fat Greek yogurt
- 1 tbsp olive oil or butter for cooking
- Fresh berries (optional)
- Salt to taste

Directions

1. In a bowl, whisk together the almond flour, eggs, almond milk, baking powder, vanilla extract, and a pinch of salt.
2. Heat the olive oil or butter in a non-stick skillet over medium heat.
3. Pour small portions of the batter into the skillet to form pancakes.
4. Cook until bubbles form on the surface, then flip and cook until golden brown.
5. Serve the pancakes topped with Greek yogurt and fresh berries if desired.

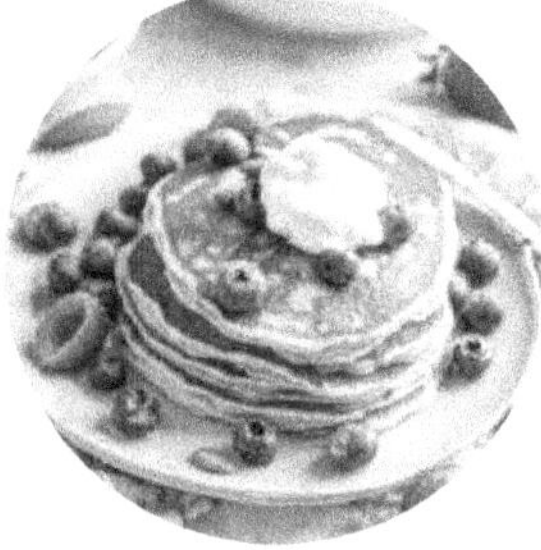

Ingredient Tips:

- Almond Flour: Low in carbohydrates and high in healthy fats and protein, making it a great choice for managing blood sugar levels.
- Greek Yogurt: Adds protein and creaminess, helping to keep you full and satisfied.

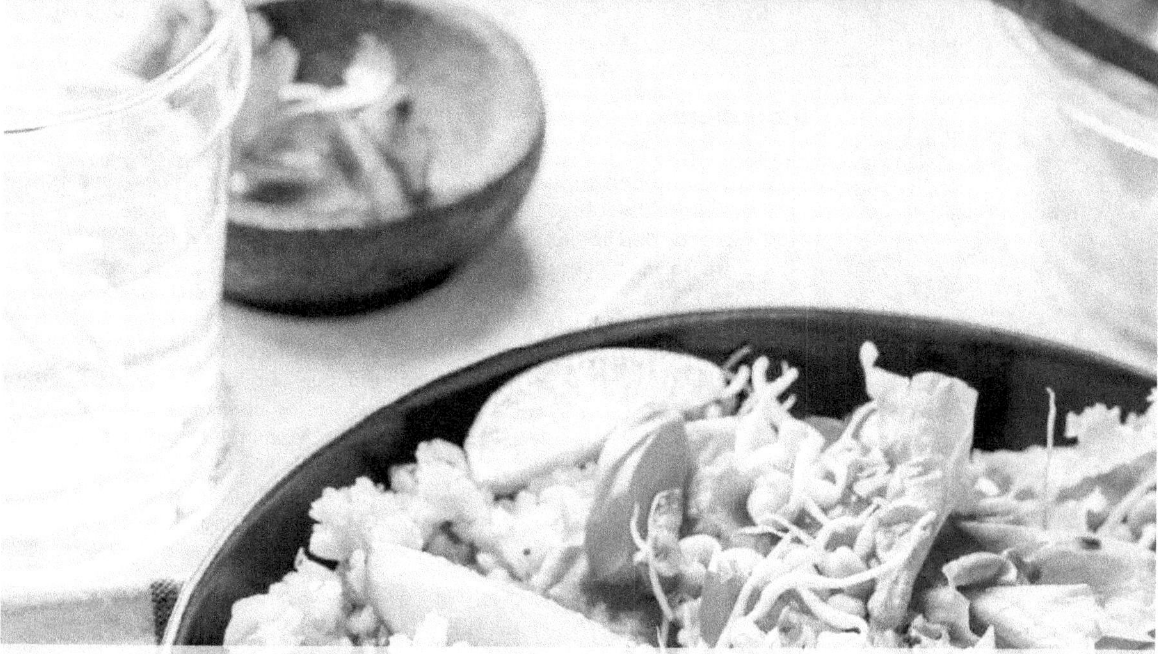

Chapter Six

Lunch Recipes

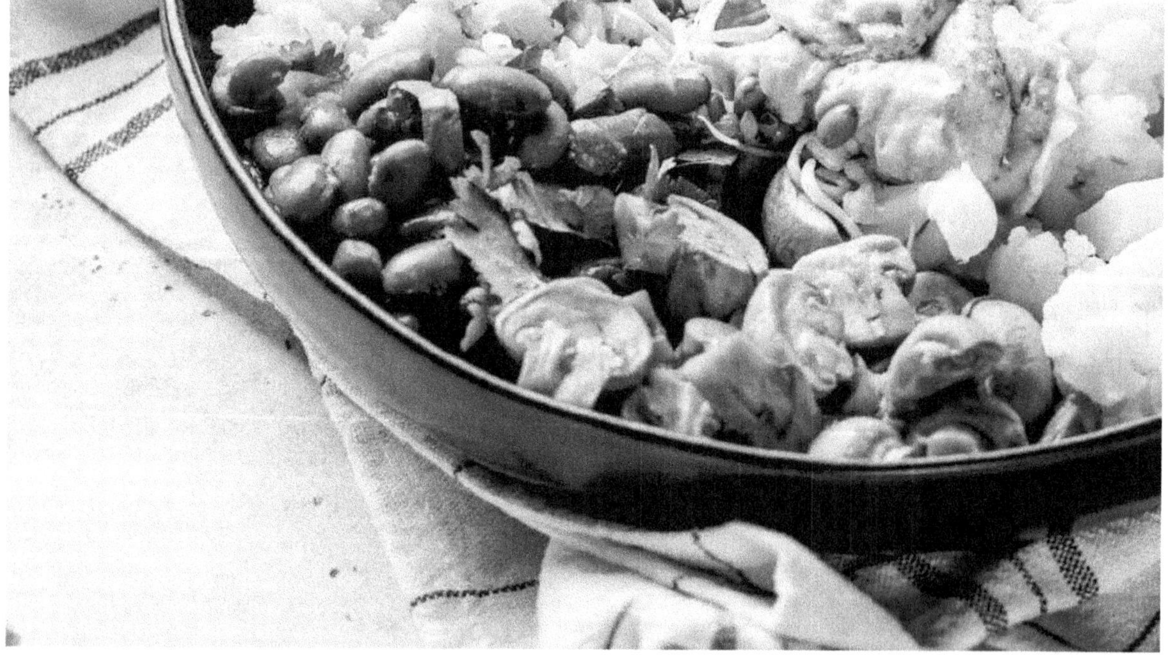

Spinach and Feta Stuffed Peppers

Flavorful and nutritious stuffed bell peppers filled with a spinach and feta mixture, perfect for a light and satisfying lunch.

Servings: 2 | Prep Time: 10 mins | Cook Time: 25 mins | Carbs per Serving: 12g

NUTRIENT CONTENT (PER SERVING):

- Calories: 180
- Total Fat: 11g
- Protein: 7g
- Carbohydrates: 12g
- Sugars: 6g
- Fiber: 4g
- Sodium: 300mg

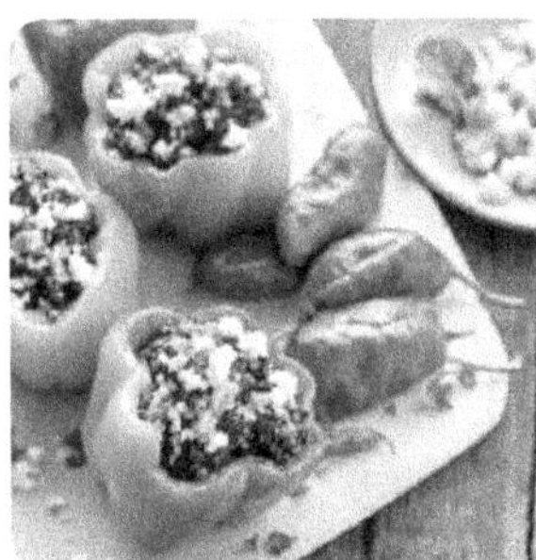

Ingredients

- 2 large bell peppers, halved and seeded
- 2 cups fresh spinach, chopped
- 1/2 cup crumbled feta cheese
- 1/4 cup red onion, diced
- 1 tbsp olive oil
- 1 clove garlic, minced
- 1/4 tsp black pepper

Directions

1. Preheat the oven to 375°F (190°C).
2. In a large skillet, heat the olive oil over medium heat.
3. Add the garlic and red onion and sauté until fragrant and softened.
4. Add the chopped spinach and cook until wilted.
5. Remove from heat and stir in the crumbled feta cheese and black.
6. Stuff the bell pepper halves with the spinach and feta mixture.
7. Place the stuffed peppers on a baking sheet and bake for 20-25 minutes, or until the peppers are tender.
8. Serve hot.

Ingredient Tips:

- Bell Peppers: Low in calories and high in vitamins A and C, making them a nutritious and fiber-rich choice.
- Spinach: Provides fiber and essential nutrients, aiding in blood sugar control.

Baked Salmon with Asparagus

A simple and elegant baked salmon dish served with tender asparagus, perfect for a nutritious and satisfying lunch.

Servings: 2 | Prep Time: 10 mins | Cook Time: 20 mins | Carbs per Serving: 7g

NUTRIENT CONTENT (PER SERVING):

- Calories: 300
- Total Fat: 18g
- Protein: 28g
- Carbohydrates: 7g
- Sugars: 2g
- Fiber: 3g
- Sodium: 200mg

Ingredients

- 2 salmon fillets (4 oz each)
- 1 bunch asparagus, trimmed
- 2 tbsp olive oil
- 1 lemon, sliced
- 1 clove garlic, minced
- Salt and pepper to taste

Directions

1. Preheat the oven to 400°F (200°C).
2. Place the salmon fillets on a baking sheet lined with parchment paper.
3. Arrange the asparagus around the salmon.
4. Drizzle olive oil over the salmon and asparagus.
5. Sprinkle minced garlic, salt, and pepper over the salmon and asparagus.
6. Place lemon slices on top of the salmon.
7. Bake for 15-20 minutes, or until the salmon is cooked through and the asparagus is tender.
8. Serve hot.

Ingredient Tips:

- Salmon: High in omega-3 fatty acids and protein, promoting heart health and blood sugar control.
- Asparagus: Low in calories and rich in fiber, vitamins, and minerals.

Tuna and Avocado Salad

A quick and easy tuna salad with avocado, fresh greens, and a light lemon dressing.

Servings: 2 | Prep Time: 10 mins | Cook Time: 0 mins | Carbs per Serving: 7g

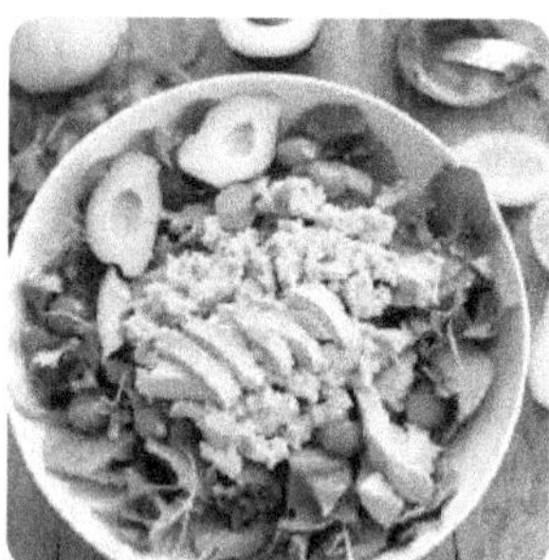

Ingredients

- 1 can tuna in water, drained
- 1/2 avocado, diced
- 2 cups mixed greens (spinach, arugula, lettuce)
- 1/2 cup cherry tomatoes, halved
- 1/4 cup red onion, thinly sliced
- 1 tbsp olive oil
- 1 tbsp lemon juice
- Salt and pepper to taste

Directions

1. In a large bowl, combine the mixed greens, cherry tomatoes, and red onion.
2. Add the drained tuna and diced avocado on top.
3. Drizzle with olive oil and lemon juice.
4. Toss gently to combine.
5. Season with salt and pepper to taste and serve.

Ingredient Tips:

- Tuna: High in protein and omega-3 fatty acids, which help to reduce inflammation and improve heart health.
- Avocado: Provides healthy fats and fiber, aiding in satiety and blood sugar control.

Chickpea and Vegetable Stir-Fry

A vibrant and nutritious stir-fry with chickpeas and fresh vegetables, perfect for a quick and satisfying lunch.

Servings: 2 | Prep Time: 10 mins | Cook Time: 10 mins | Carbs per Serving: 22g

Ingredients

- 1 can chickpeas, drained and rinsed
- 1 cup broccoli florets
- 1 bell pepper, sliced
- 1 carrot, sliced
- 1/2 cup snap peas
- 2 tbsp olive oil
- 2 tbsp soy sauce (low sodium)
- 1 tsp ginger, minced
- 1 clove garlic, minced
- Salt and pepper to taste

Directions

1. In a large skillet, heat the olive oil over medium-high heat.
2. Add the ginger and garlic and sauté until fragrant.
3. Add the broccoli, bell pepper, carrot, and snap peas and cook until tender-crisp.
4. Add the chickpeas and soy sauce and stir to combine.
5. Cook for another 2-3 minutes, or until heated through.
6. Season with salt and pepper to taste and serve hot.

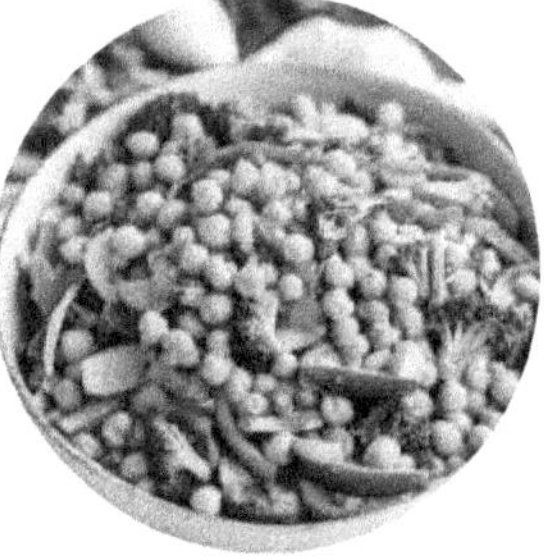

Ingredient Tips:

- Chickpeas: High in protein and fiber, making them an excellent option for managing blood sugar levels.
- Vegetables: Adding a variety of vegetables increases the fiber content, aiding in digestion and blood sugar control.

Grilled Chicken and Avocado Salad

A refreshing and protein-packed salad with grilled chicken, avocado, and fresh greens, perfect for a light yet satisfying lunch.

Servings: 2 | Prep Time: 10 mins | Cook Time: 10 mins | Carbs per Serving: 8g

NUTRIENT CONTENT (PER SERVING):

- Calories: 320
- Total Fat: 20g
- Protein: 28g
- Carbohydrates: 8g
- Sugars: 3g
- Fiber: 5g
- Sodium: 220mg

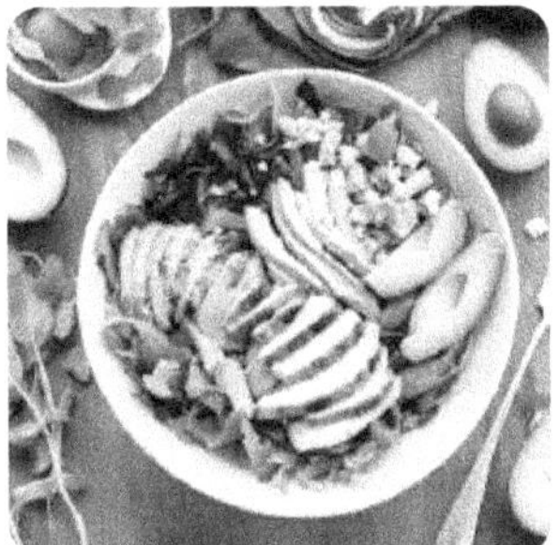

Ingredients

- 1 grilled chicken breast, sliced
- 1/2 avocado, diced
- 2 cups mixed greens (spinach, arugula, lettuce)
- 1/2 cup cherry tomatoes, halved
- 1/4 cup cucumber, sliced
- 1 tbsp olive oil
- 1 tbsp lemon juice
- Salt and pepper to taste

Directions

1. In a large bowl, combine the mixed greens, cherry tomatoes, and cucumber.
2. Add the grilled chicken slices and diced avocado on top.
3. Drizzle with olive oil and lemon juice.
4. Toss gently to combine.
5. Season with salt and pepper to taste and serve.

Ingredient Tips:

- Grilled Chicken: High in protein, helping to keep you full and manage blood sugar levels.
- Avocado: Provides healthy fats and fiber, aiding in satiety and blood sugar control.

Quinoa and Black Bean Salad

A hearty and nutritious quinoa and black bean salad with fresh vegetables and a tangy lime dressing.

Servings: 3 | Prep Time: 15 mins | Cook Time: 15 mins | Carbs per Serving: 34g

NUTRIENT CONTENT (PER SERVING):

- Calories: 280
- Total Fat: 12g
- Protein: 9g
- Carbohydrates: 34g
- Sugars: 3g
- Fiber: 8g
- Sodium: 250mg

Ingredients

- 1 cup cooked quinoa
- 1 cup black beans, drained and rinsed
- 1/2 cup corn kernels
- 1/2 cup diced bell peppers
- 1/4 cup red onion, diced
- 1/4 cup chopped cilantro
- 2 tbsp olive oil
- 2 tbsp lime juice
- Salt and pepper to taste

Directions

1. In a large bowl, combine the cooked quinoa, black beans, corn, bell peppers, red onion, and cilantro.
2. In a small bowl, whisk together the olive oil, lime juice, salt, and pepper.
3. Pour the dressing over the salad and toss to combine.
4. Serve chilled or at room temperature.

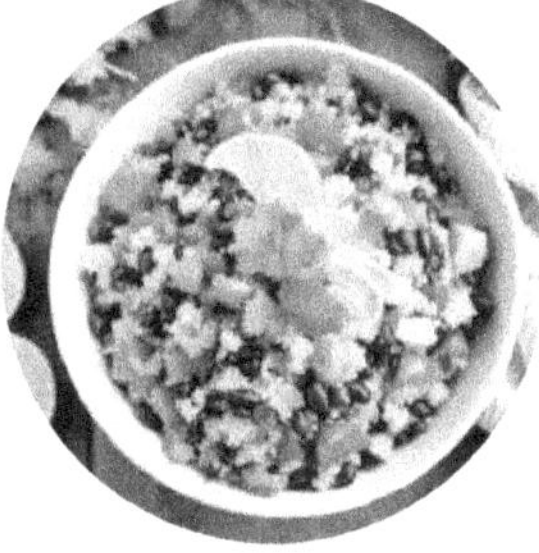

Ingredient Tips:

- Quinoa: A whole grain high in protein and fiber, helping to maintain steady blood sugar levels.
- Black Beans: High in protein and fiber, making them an excellent option for managing blood sugar levels.

Turkey and Spinach Wrap

A delicious and easy-to-make turkey wrap with fresh spinach, avocado, and a tangy yogurt sauce.

Servings: 1 | Prep Time: 10 mins | Cook Time: 0 mins | Carbs per Serving :28g

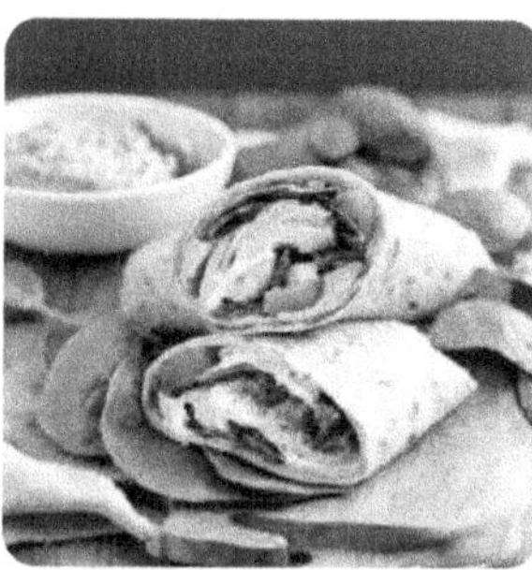

Ingredients

- 1 whole grain tortilla
- 3 slices deli turkey breast
- 1/2 avocado, sliced
- 1 cup fresh spinach
- 2 tbsp plain Greek yogurt
- 1 tsp Dijon mustard
- Salt and pepper to taste

Directions

1. In a small bowl, mix the Greek yogurt and Dijon mustard.
2. Spread the yogurt mixture onto the tortilla.
3. Layer the turkey slices, avocado, and spinach on top.
4. Roll up the tortilla tightly and slice in half.
5. Serve immediately.

Ingredient Tips:

- Turkey Breast: Low in fat and high in protein, helping to keep you full and manage blood sugar levels.
- Spinach: Low in carbohydrates and high in fiber, making it a great choice for managing blood sugar levels.

Lentil and Vegetable Soup

A warm and comforting lentil soup packed with fresh vegetables for a nutritious and filling lunch.

Servings: 4 | Prep Time: 15 mins | Cook Time: 25 mins | Carbs per Serving: 25g

Ingredients

- 1 cup dried lentils, rinsed
- 1 carrot, diced
- 1 celery stalk, diced
- 1 onion, diced
- 2 cups spinach, chopped
- 1 can diced tomatoes (14.5 oz)
- 4 cups vegetable broth
- 2 tbsp olive oil
- 2 cloves garlic, minced
- 1 tsp cumin
- 1 tsp paprika
- Salt and pepper to taste

Directions

1. In a large pot, heat the olive oil over medium heat.
2. Add the garlic, onion, carrot, and celery and sauté until softened.
3. Add the cumin and paprika and cook for another minute.
4. Add the lentils, diced tomatoes, and vegetable broth.
5. Bring to a boil, then reduce heat and simmer for 20-25 minutes, or until lentils are tender.
6. Stir in the chopped spinach and cook until wilted.
7. Season with salt and pepper to taste and serve hot.

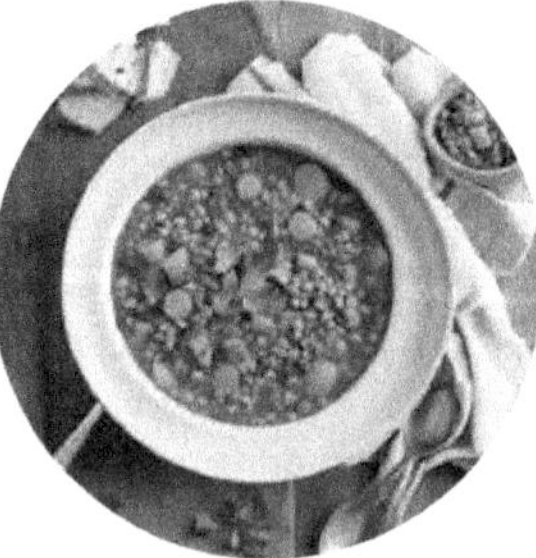

Ingredient Tips:

- Lentils: High in protein and fiber, making them an excellent option for managing blood sugar levels.
- Vegetables: Adding a variety of vegetables increases the fiber content, aiding in digestion and blood sugar control.

Chickpea and Spinach Curry

A flavorful and protein-rich chickpea and spinach curry served with a side of brown rice for a balanced and satisfying lunch.

Servings: 2 | Prep Time: 15 mins | Cook Time: 15 mins | Carbs per Serving :45g

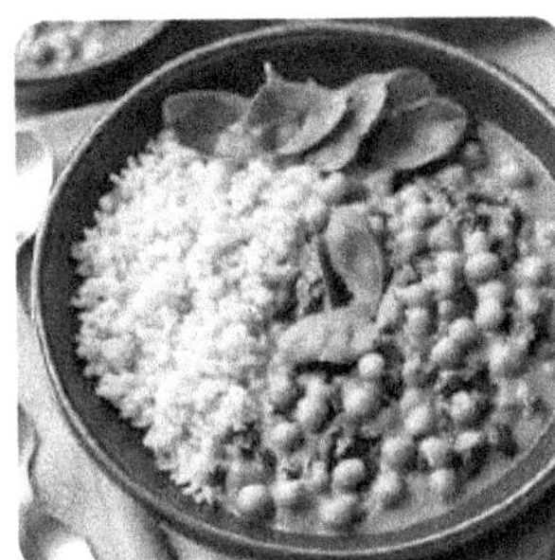

Ingredients

- 1 can chickpeas, drained and rinsed
- 2 cups fresh spinach, chopped
- 1 cup canned diced tomatoes
- 1/2 cup coconut milk
- 1 onion, diced
- 2 cloves garlic, minced
- 1 tbsp olive oil
- 1 tsp curry powder
- 1/2 tsp cumin
- Salt and pepper to taste
- 1 cup cooked brown rice

Directions

1. In a large skillet, heat the olive oil over medium heat.
2. Add the garlic and onion and sauté until softened.
3. Add the curry powder and cumin and cook for another minute.
4. Add the diced tomatoes and coconut milk and bring to a simmer.
5. Stir in the chickpeas and chopped spinach.
6. Simmer for 10-15 minutes, or until the spinach is wilted and the chickpeas are heated through.
7. Season with salt and pepper to taste.
8. Serve the curry over a bed of cooked brown rice.

Ingredient Tips:

- Chickpeas: High in protein and fiber, helping to manage blood sugar levels.
- Spinach: Low in carbohydrates and high in fiber and essential nutrients.

Turkey and Vegetable Lettuce Wraps

Light and refreshing lettuce wraps filled with lean turkey and fresh vegetables, perfect for a quick and healthy lunch.

Servings: 4 | Prep Time: 10 mins | Cook Time: 15 mins | Carbs per Serving: 10g

Ingredients

- 1 lb ground turkey
- 1 cup shredded carrots
- 1 bell pepper, diced
- 1/2 cup diced water chestnuts
- 1/4 cup green onions, sliced
- 1 tbsp olive oil
- 2 tbsp soy sauce (low sodium)
- 1 tsp ginger, minced
- 1 clove garlic, minced
- 8 large lettuce leaves (Bibb or Romaine)
- Salt and pepper to taste

Directions

1. In a large skillet, heat the olive oil over medium heat.
2. Add the garlic and ginger and sauté until fragrant.
3. Add the ground turkey and cook until browned.
4. Stir in the soy sauce, shredded carrots, bell pepper, water chestnuts, and green onions.
5. Cook until the vegetables are tender and the turkey is fully cooked.
6. Season with salt and pepper to taste.
7. Spoon the turkey and vegetable mixture into the lettuce leaves and serve.

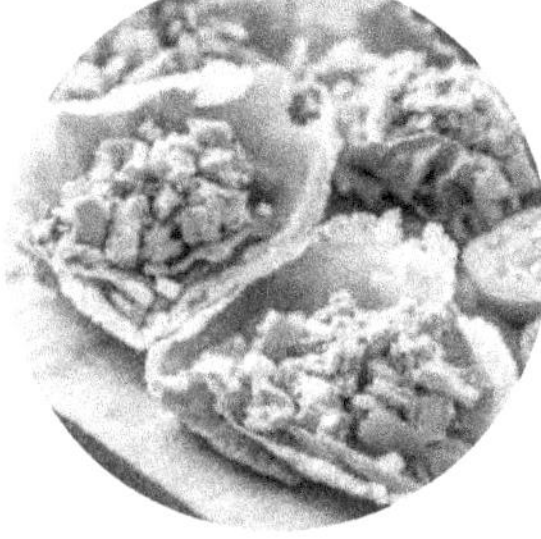

Ingredient Tips:

- Ground Turkey: Lean and high in protein, helping to keep you full and manage blood sugar levels.
- Lettuce: Low in calories and carbohydrates, making it a great alternative to bread or wraps.

Cauliflower Rice and Shrimp Stir-Fry

A low-carb and flavorful stir-fry with cauliflower rice, shrimp, and fresh vegetables, perfect for a satisfying and nutritious lunch.

Servings: 3 | Prep Time: 10 mins | Cook Time: 15 mins | Carbs per Serving :15g

NUTRIENT CONTENT (PER SERVING):

- Calories: 280
- Total Fat: 12g
- Protein: 26g
- Carbohydrates: 15g
- Sugars: 6g
- Fiber: 6g
- Sodium: 500mg

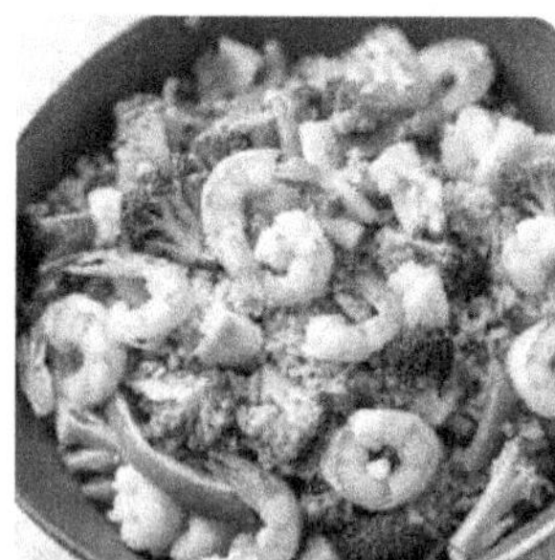

Ingredients

- 1 lb shrimp, peeled and deveined
- 4 cups cauliflower rice
- 1 cup snap peas
- 1 bell pepper, sliced
- 1 carrot, sliced
- 2 tbsp olive oil
- 2 cloves garlic, minced
- 1 tbsp soy sauce (low sodium)
- 1 tsp sesame oil
- Salt and pepper to taste

Directions

1. In a large skillet, heat 1 tbsp of olive oil over medium-high heat.
2. Add the shrimp and cook until pink and cooked through, about 3-4 minutes. Remove and set aside.
3. In the same skillet, heat the remaining olive oil.
4. Add the garlic and sauté until fragrant.
5. Add the cauliflower rice, snap peas, bell pepper, and carrot and cook until tender-crisp.
6. Stir in the cooked shrimp, soy sauce, and sesame oil.
7. Season with salt and pepper to taste and serve hot.

Ingredient Tips:

- Shrimp: Low in calories and high in protein, making it a great choice for managing blood sugar levels.
- Cauliflower Rice: A low-carb alternative to regular rice, helping to keep carbohydrate intake low.

Chicken and Broccoli Stir-Fry

A simple and healthy chicken and broccoli stir-fry with a savory soy sauce glaze, perfect for a quick and balanced lunch.

Servings: 3 | Prep Time: 10 mins | Cook Time: 15 mins | Carbs per Serving: 12g

NUTRIENT CONTENT (PER SERVING):

- Calories: 260
- Total Fat: 12g
- Protein: 30g
- Carbohydrates: 12g
- Sugars: 6g
- Fiber: 4g
- Sodium: 450mg

Ingredients

- 1 lb chicken breast, sliced into thin strips
- 2 cups broccoli florets
- 1 bell pepper, sliced
- 1/4 cup onion, sliced
- 2 tbsp olive oil
- 2 tbsp soy sauce (low sodium)
- 1 tbsp oyster sauce
- 1 clove garlic, minced
- Salt and pepper to taste

Directions

1. In a large skillet, heat 1 tbsp of olive oil over medium-high heat.
2. Add the chicken strips and cook until browned and cooked through. Remove and set aside.
3. In the same skillet, heat the remaining olive oil.
4. Add the garlic and sauté until fragrant.
5. Add the broccoli, bell pepper, and onion and cook until tender-crisp.
6. Stir in the cooked chicken, soy sauce, and oyster sauce.
7. Season with salt and pepper to taste and serve hot.

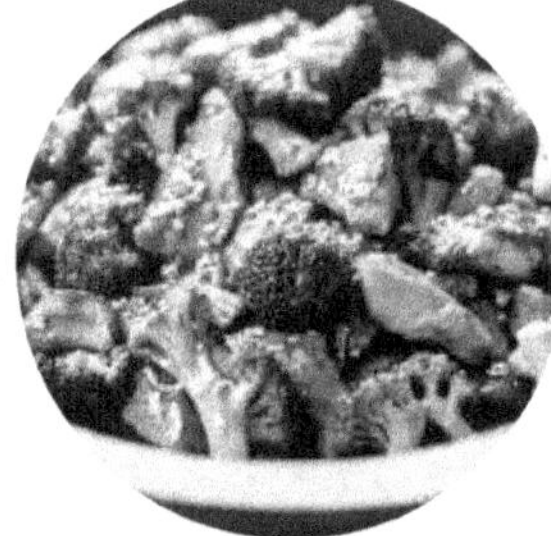

Ingredient Tips:

- Chicken Breast: Lean and high in protein, helping to keep you full and manage blood sugar levels.
- Broccoli: Low in calories and high in fiber, making it a great vegetable for blood sugar control.

Lentil and Vegetable Stew

A hearty and nutritious lentil stew with a variety of vegetables, perfect for a comforting and satisfying lunch.

Servings: 4 | Prep Time: 10 mins | Cook Time: 30 mins | Carbs per Serving :30g

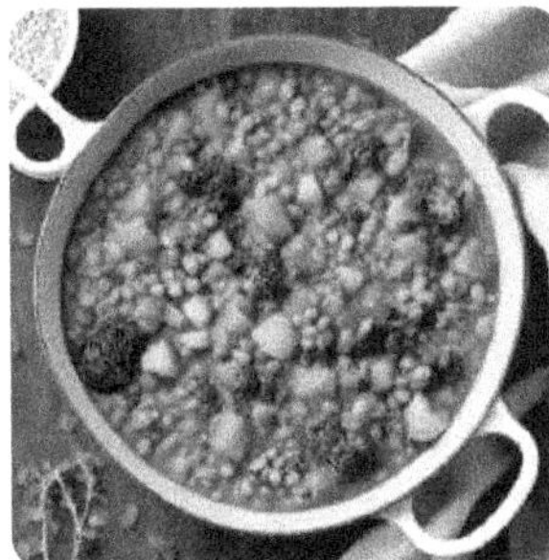

Ingredients

- 1 cup dried lentils, rinsed
- 1 cup diced tomatoes
- 1 carrot, diced
- 1 celery stalk, diced
- 1 onion, diced
- 2 cloves garlic, minced
- 4 cups vegetable broth (low sodium)
- 1 tbsp olive oil
- 1 tsp cumin
- 1 tsp paprika
- Salt and pepper to taste

Directions

1. In a large pot, heat the olive oil over medium heat.
2. Add the garlic and onion and sauté until softened.
3. Add the carrot and celery and cook for a few more minutes.
4. Stir in the cumin and paprika and cook for another minute.
5. Add the lentils, diced tomatoes, and vegetable broth.
6. Bring to a boil, then reduce the heat and simmer for 25-30 minutes, or until the lentils are tender.
7. Season with salt and pepper to taste and serve hot.

Ingredient Tips:

- Lentils: High in protein and fiber, making them excellent for managing blood sugar levels.
- Vegetable Broth: Use low-sodium broth to keep the sodium content in check.

Tofu and Vegetable Stir-Fry

A quick and easy tofu stir-fry with a variety of fresh vegetables, perfect for a nutritious and balanced lunch.

Servings: 3 | Prep Time: 10 mins | Cook Time: 15 mins | Carbs per Serving: 10g

Ingredients

- 1 block firm tofu, cubed
- 1 cup snap peas
- 1 bell pepper, sliced
- 1 carrot, sliced
- 2 tbsp olive oil
- 2 tbsp soy sauce (low sodium)
- 1 tbsp sesame oil
- 1 clove garlic, minced
- Salt and pepper to taste

Directions

1. In a large skillet, heat 1 tbsp of olive oil over medium-high heat.
2. Add the tofu cubes and cook until golden brown on all sides. Remove and set aside.
3. In the same skillet, heat the remaining olive oil.
4. Add the garlic and sauté until fragrant.
5. Add the snap peas, bell pepper, and carrot and cook until tender-crisp.
6. Stir in the cooked tofu, soy sauce, and sesame oil.
7. Season with salt and pepper to taste and serve hot.

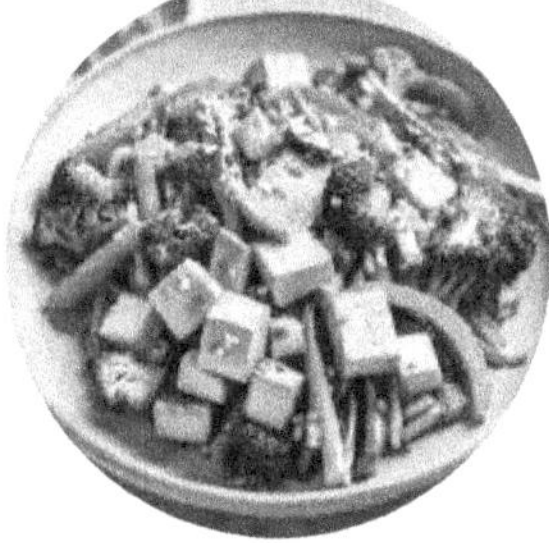

Ingredient Tips:

- Tofu: A plant-based protein that helps keep you full and manage blood sugar levels.
- Snap Peas: Low in calories and high in fiber, making them a great vegetable for blood sugar control.

Turkey and Avocado Wrap

A simple and delicious turkey and avocado wrap with fresh vegetables, perfect for a quick and healthy lunch.

NUTRIENT CONTENT (PER SERVING):
- Calories: 250
- Total Fat: 12g
- Protein: 16g
- Carbohydrates: 20g
- Sugars: 2g
- Fiber: 5g
- Sodium: 400mg

Servings: 4 | Prep Time: 10 mins | Cook Time: 0 mins | Carbs per Serving :20g

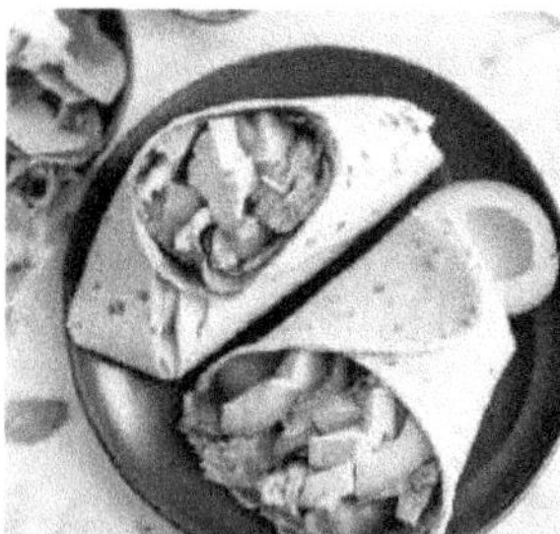

Ingredients

- 4 whole grain tortillas
- 1/2 lb sliced turkey breast
- 1 avocado, sliced
- 1/2 cup shredded lettuce
- 1/2 cup cherry tomatoes, halved
- 1/4 cup red onion, thinly sliced
- 2 tbsp olive oil
- 1 tbsp lime juice
- Salt and pepper to taste

Directions

1. Lay the tortillas flat on a clean surface.
2. Divide the sliced turkey breast evenly among the tortillas.
3. Top with avocado slices, shredded lettuce, cherry tomatoes, and red onion.
4. In a small bowl, whisk together the olive oil, lime juice, salt, and pepper.
5. Drizzle the dressing over the fillings.
6. Roll up the tortillas and serve.

Ingredient Tips:

- Turkey Breast: Lean and high in protein, helping to keep you full and manage blood sugar levels.
- Whole Grain Tortillas: Provide complex carbohydrates and fiber, aiding in blood sugar control.

Zucchini Noodles with Pesto & Chicken

A low-carb and flavorful dish with zucchini noodles, homemade pesto, and grilled chicken, perfect for a light and nutritious lunch.

NUTRIENT CONTENT (PER SERVING):
- Calories: 320
- Total Fat: 20g
- Protein: 26g
- Carbohydrates: 10g
- Sugars: 4g
- Fiber: 4g
- Sodium: 300mg

Servings: 2 | Prep Time: 10 mins | Cook Time: 15 mins | Carbs per Serving: 10g

Ingredients

- 2 large zucchini, spiralized
- 2 chicken breasts
- 1/2 cup basil pesto
- 1/2 cup cherry tomatoes, halved
- 2 tbsp olive oil
- Salt and pepper to taste
- Fresh basil for garnish

Directions

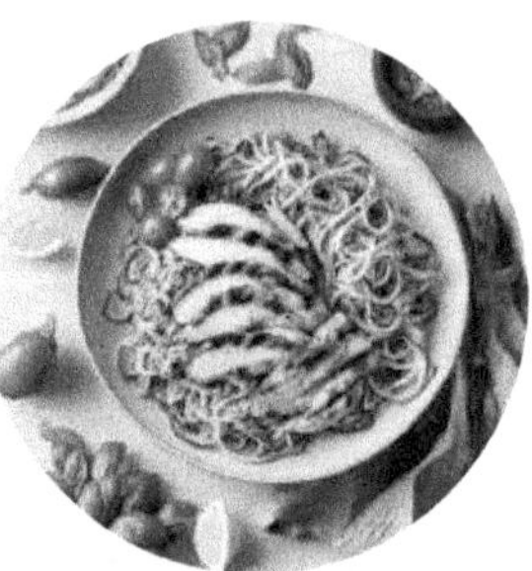

1. Season the chicken breasts with salt and pepper.
2. Grill the chicken over medium heat until cooked through, about 5-7 minutes per side. Let rest, then slice.
3. In a large skillet, heat the olive oil over medium heat.
4. Add the spiralized zucchini and cook until just tender, about 2-3 minutes.
5. Remove from heat and toss with basil pesto.
6. Top with sliced grilled chicken and cherry tomatoes.
7. Garnish with fresh basil and serve.

Ingredient Tips:

- Zucchini Noodles: A low-carb alternative to pasta, helping to keep carbohydrate intake low.
- Pesto: Made with healthy fats from olive oil and nuts, aiding in blood sugar control.

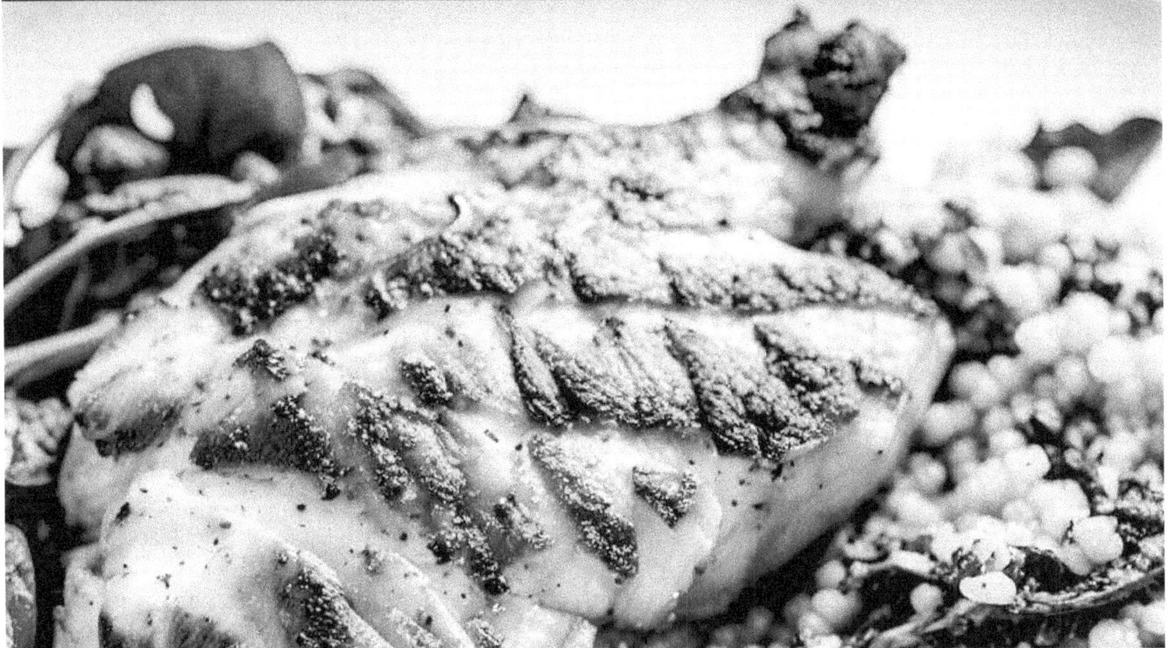

Chapter Seven

Dinner Recipes

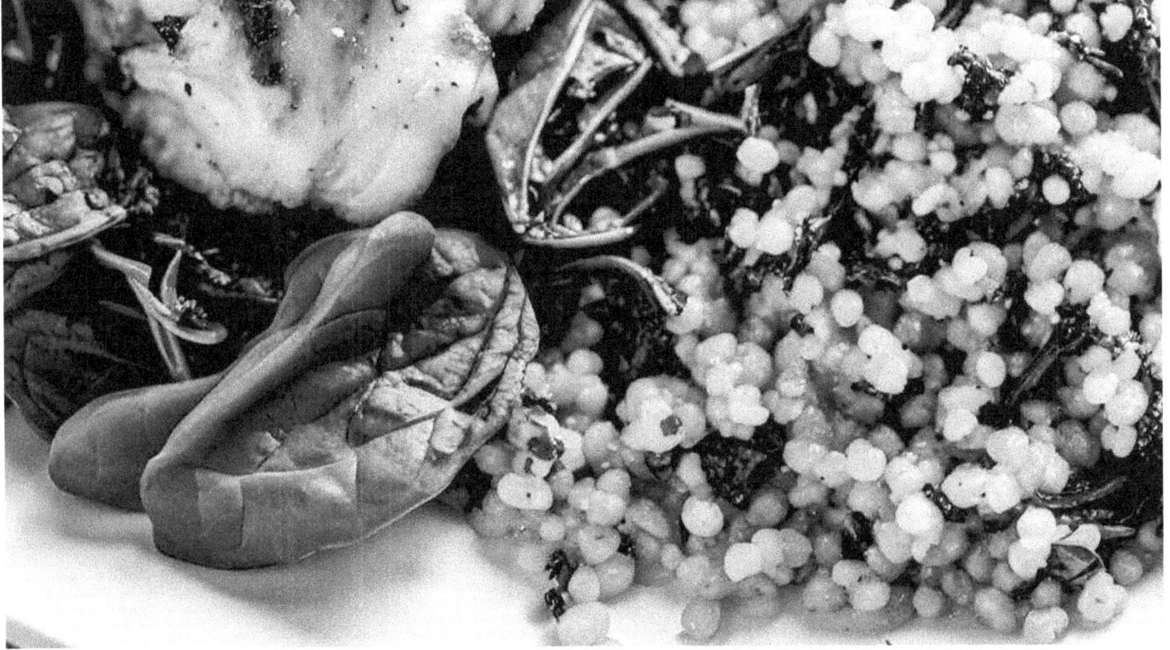

Baked Salmon with Avocado Salsa

A simple yet flavorful baked salmon topped with a fresh avocado salsa, perfect for a healthy and satisfying dinner.

Servings: 4 | Prep Time: 10 mins | Cook Time:15 mins | Carbs per Serving :8g

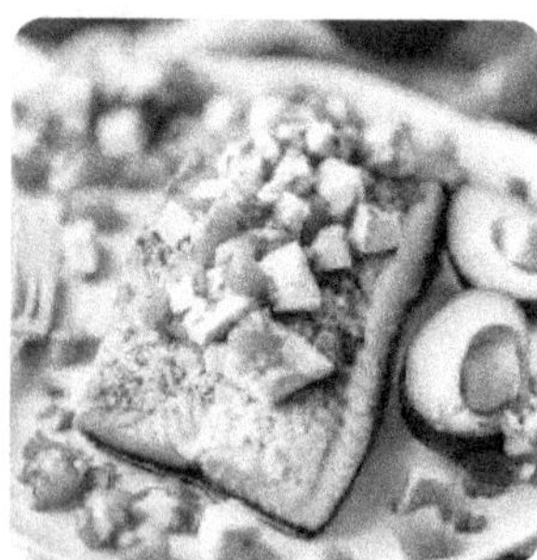

Ingredients

- 4 salmon fillets
- 1 avocado, diced
- 1 cup cherry tomatoes, halved
- 1/4 cup red onion, diced
- 2 tbsp olive oil
- 1 tbsp lime juice
- Salt and pepper to taste

Directions

1. Preheat the oven to 400°F (200°C).
2. Season the salmon fillets with salt and pepper and place them on a baking sheet.
3. Bake for 12-15 minutes or until the salmon is cooked through.
4. In a bowl, combine the diced avocado, cherry tomatoes, red onion, olive oil, and lime juice.
5. Season the avocado salsa with salt and pepper.
6. Top each salmon fillet with the avocado salsa before serving.

Ingredient Tips:

- Salmon: Rich in omega-3 fatty acids, which help manage blood sugar levels and promote heart health.
- Avocado: Provides healthy fats and fiber, aiding in blood sugar control.

Grilled Chicken with Quinoa & Spinach

A protein-packed grilled chicken served with quinoa and sautéed spinach, perfect for a balanced and nutritious dinner.

Servings: 4 | Prep Time: 10 mins | Cook Time: 15 mins | Carbs per Serving: 25g

Ingredients

- 4 chicken breasts
- 1 cup quinoa, cooked
- 4 cups fresh spinach
- 2 tbsp olive oil
- 2 cloves garlic, minced
- Salt and pepper to taste

Directions

1. Season the chicken breasts with salt and pepper.
2. Grill the chicken over medium heat until cooked through, about 5-7 minutes per side.
3. In a large skillet, heat the olive oil over medium heat.
4. Add the garlic and sauté until fragrant.
5. Add the spinach and cook until wilted.
6. Serve the grilled chicken with quinoa and sautéed spinach.

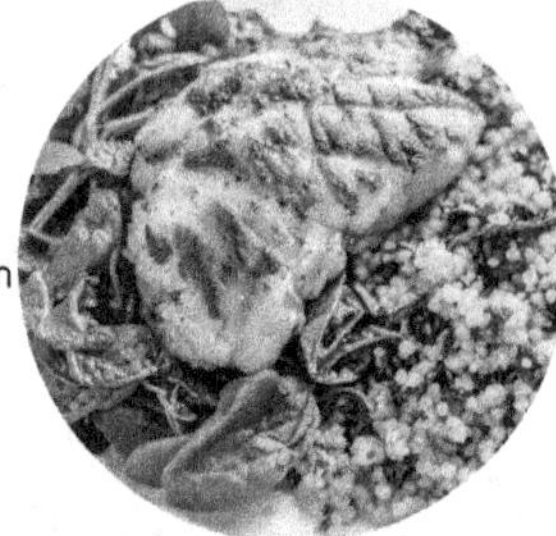

Ingredient Tips:

- Chicken Breast: Lean and high in protein, helping to keep you full and manage blood sugar levels.
- Quinoa: A high-protein grain that is also rich in fiber, helping to manage blood sugar levels.

Baked Cod with Lemon & Asparagus

A light and flavorful baked cod with lemon and asparagus, perfect for a nutritious and balanced dinner.

Servings: 4 | Prep Time: 10 mins | Cook Time:15 mins | Carbs per Serving :5g

NUTRIENT CONTENT (PER SERVING):

- Calories: 220
- Total Fat: 10g
- Protein: 30g
- Carbohydrates: 5g
- Sugars: 2g
- Fiber: 2g
- Sodium: 150mg

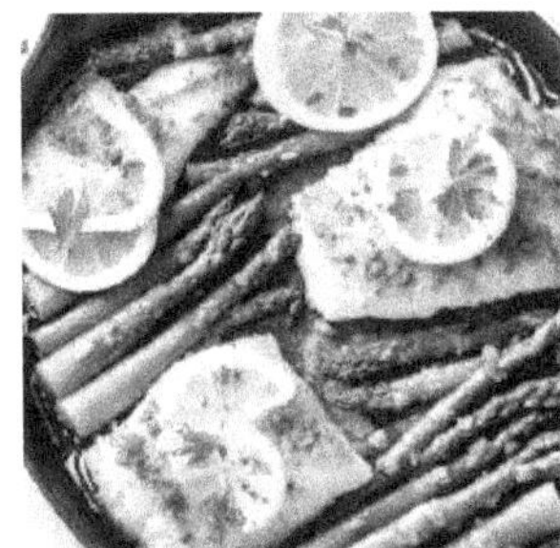

Ingredients

- 4 cod fillets
- 1 bunch asparagus, trimmed
- 2 tbsp olive oil
- 1 lemon, sliced
- 2 cloves garlic, minced
- Salt and pepper to taste

Directions

1. Preheat the oven to 400°F (200°C).
2. Place the cod fillets and asparagus on a baking sheet.
3. Drizzle with olive oil and top with lemon slices and minced garlic.
4. Season with salt and pepper.
5. Bake for 12-15 minutes or until the cod is cooked through and the asparagus is tender.
6. Serve immediately.

Ingredient Tips:

- Cod: A lean source of protein that is low in calories and high in nutrients.
- Asparagus: Low in calories and high in fiber, making it a great vegetable for blood sugar control.

Beef and Vegetable Skewers

Flavorful beef and vegetable skewers, perfect for a delicious and balanced dinner

Servings: 4 | Prep Time: 15 mins | Cook Time: 10 mins | Carbs per Serving: 8g

NUTRIENT CONTENT (PER SERVING):

- Calories: 320
- Total Fat: 18g
- Protein: 30g
- Carbohydrates: 8g
- Sugars: 4g
- Fiber: 2g
- Sodium: 200mg

Ingredients

- 1 lb beef sirloin, cut into cubes
- 1 bell pepper, cut into squares
- 1 zucchini, sliced
- 1 red onion, cut into squares
- 2 tbsp olive oil
- 1 tbsp balsamic vinegar
- 1 tsp dried oregano
- Salt and pepper to taste

Directions

1. Preheat the grill to medium-high heat.
2. In a bowl, combine the olive oil, balsamic vinegar, dried oregano, salt, and pepper.
3. Thread the beef, bell pepper, zucchini, and red onion onto skewers.
4. Brush the skewers with the olive oil mixture.
5. Grill the skewers for 8-10 minutes, turning occasionally, until the beef is cooked to your liking and the vegetables are tender.
6. Serve immediately.

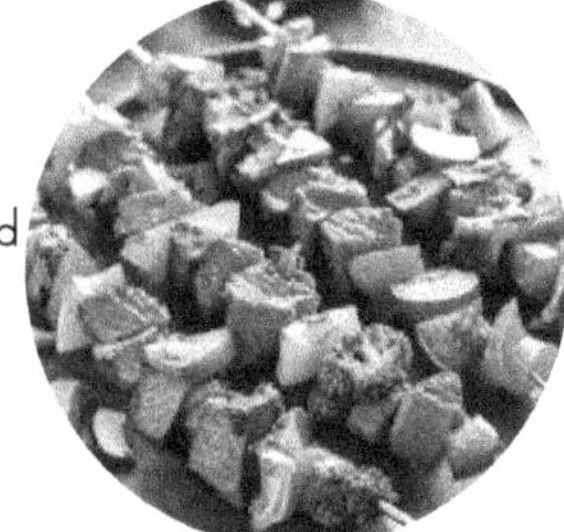

Ingredient Tips:

- Beef Sirloin: A lean cut of beef that provides high-quality protein.
- Vegetables: Adding a variety of vegetables increases the fiber content, which helps manage blood sugar levels.

Shrimp and Vegetable Stir-Fry

A quick and easy shrimp stir-fry with a variety of fresh vegetables, perfect for a healthy and balanced dinner.

Servings: 4 | Prep Time: 10 mins | Cook Time:15 mins | Carbs per Serving :12g

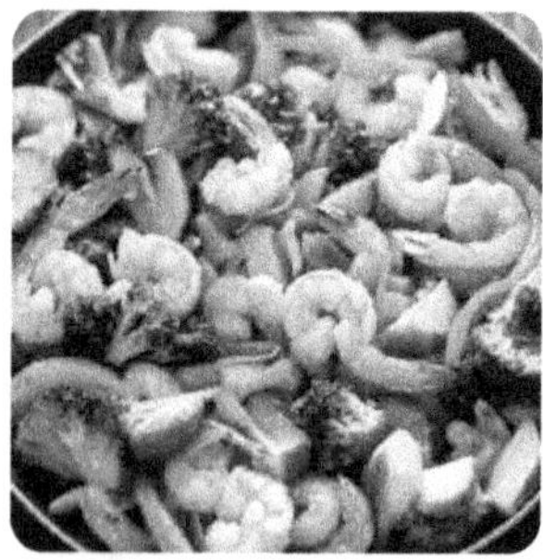

Ingredients

- 1 lb shrimp, peeled and deveined
- 1 cup broccoli florets
- 1 bell pepper, sliced
- 1 carrot, sliced
- 2 tbsp olive oil
- 2 tbsp soy sauce (low sodium)
- 1 tbsp sesame oil
- 1 clove garlic, minced
- Salt and pepper to taste

Directions

1. In a large skillet, heat 1 tbsp of olive oil over medium-high heat.
2. Add the shrimp and cook until pink and opaque. Remove and set aside.
3. In the same skillet, heat the remaining olive oil.
4. Add the garlic and sauté until fragrant.
5. Add the broccoli, bell pepper, and carrot and cook until tender-crisp.
6. Stir in the cooked shrimp, soy sauce, and sesame oil.
7. Season with salt and pepper to taste and serve hot.

Ingredient Tips:

- Shrimp: Low in calories and high in protein, making them a great option for blood sugar control.
- Broccoli: Low in calories and high in fiber, making it a great vegetable for blood sugar control.

Turkey Meatballs with Zucchini Noodles

Delicious and tender turkey meatballs served over zucchini noodles, perfect for a low-carb and satisfying dinner.

Servings: 4 | Prep Time: 15 mins | Cook Time: 25 mins | Carbs per Serving: 15g

Ingredients

- 1 lb ground turkey
- 1 egg
- 1/4 cup grated Parmesan cheese
- 1/4 cup breadcrumbs (optional)
- 2 cloves garlic, minced
- 1 tbsp olive oil
- 2 large zucchini, spiralized
- 1 cup marinara sauce (low sodium)
- Salt and pepper to taste

Directions

1. Preheat the oven to 375°F (190°C).
2. In a bowl, combine the ground turkey, egg, Parmesan cheese, breadcrumbs, garlic, salt, and pepper.
3. Form the mixture into meatballs and place them on a baking sheet.
4. Bake for 20-25 minutes or until cooked through.
5. In a large skillet, heat the olive oil over medium heat.
6. Add the spiralized zucchini and cook until just tender, about 2-3 minutes.
7. Serve the meatballs over the zucchini noodles, topped with marinara sauce

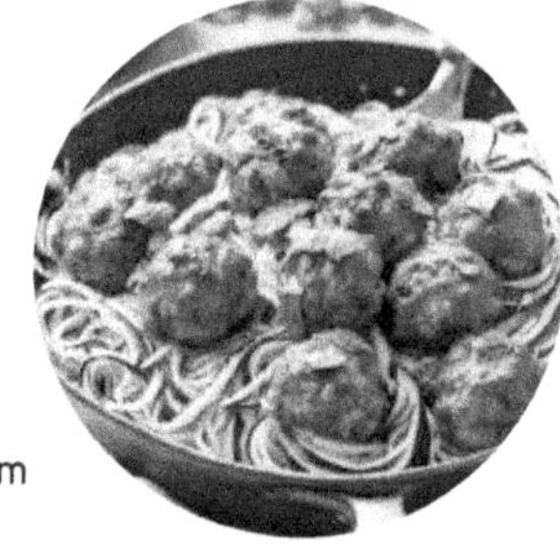

Ingredient Tips:

- Ground Turkey: Lean and high in protein, helping to keep you full and manage blood sugar levels.
- Zucchini Noodles: A low-carb alternative to pasta, helping to keep carbohydrate intake low.

Chicken and Vegetable Curry

A flavorful chicken and vegetable curry, perfect for a comforting and nutritious dinner.

Servings: 4 | Prep Time: 10 mins | Cook Time:20 mins | Carbs per Serving :15g

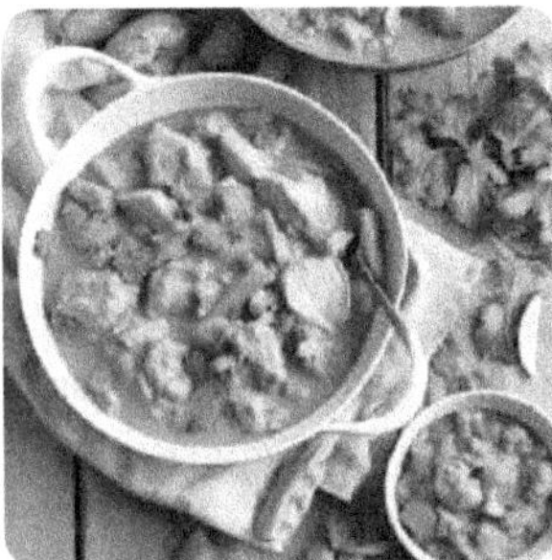

Ingredients

- 1 lb chicken breast, cut into cubes
- 1 cup cauliflower florets
- 1 cup diced tomatoes
- 1 cup coconut milk (light)
- 1 onion, diced
- 2 cloves garlic, minced
- 1 tbsp curry powder
- 1 tbsp olive oil
- Salt and pepper to taste

Directions

1. In a large pot, heat the olive oil over medium heat.
2. Add the garlic and onion and sauté until softened.
3. Add the chicken and cook until browned.
4. Stir in the curry powder and cook for another minute.
5. Add the cauliflower, diced tomatoes, and coconut milk.
6. Bring to a simmer and cook for 15-20 minutes, or until the chicken is cooked through and the vegetables are tender.
7. Season with salt and pepper to taste and serve hot.

Ingredient Tips:

- Chicken Breast: Lean and high in protein, helping to keep you full and manage blood sugar levels.
- Cauliflower: Low in calories and high in fiber, making it a great vegetable for blood sugar control.

Tofu and Vegetable Stir-Fry

A quick and easy tofu stir-fry with a variety of fresh vegetables, perfect for a healthy and balanced dinner.

Servings: 4 | Prep Time: 10 mins | Cook Time: 15 mins | Carbs per Serving: 12g

Ingredients

- 1 block firm tofu, cubed
- 1 cup snap peas
- 1 bell pepper, sliced
- 1 carrot, sliced
- 2 tbsp soy sauce (low sodium)
- 1 tbsp sesame oil
- 1 tbsp olive oil
- 1 clove garlic, minced
- Salt and pepper to taste

Directions

1. In a large skillet, heat the olive oil over medium-high heat.
2. Add the tofu and cook until golden brown on all sides. Remove and set aside.
3. In the same skillet, heat the sesame oil.
4. Add the garlic and sauté until fragrant.
5. Add the snap peas, bell pepper, and carrot and cook until tender-crisp.
6. Stir in the cooked tofu and soy sauce.
7. Season with salt and pepper to taste and serve hot.

Ingredient Tips:

- Tofu: High in protein and low in calories, making it a great option for blood sugar control.
- Snap Peas: Low in calories and high in fiber, making them a great vegetable for blood sugar control.

Baked Chicken with Brussels Sprouts

A simple and delicious baked chicken with roasted Brussels sprouts, perfect for a healthy and balanced dinner.

Servings: 4 | Prep Time: 10 mins | Cook Time:30 mins | Carbs per Serving :10g

<table>
<tr><td colspan="2">NUTRIENT CONTENT (PER SERVING):</td></tr>
<tr><td>Calories: 340</td><td>Sugars: 2g</td></tr>
<tr><td>Total Fat: 20g</td><td>Fiber: 4g</td></tr>
<tr><td>Protein: 28g</td><td>Sodium: 200mg</td></tr>
<tr><td>Carbohydrates: 10g</td><td></td></tr>
</table>

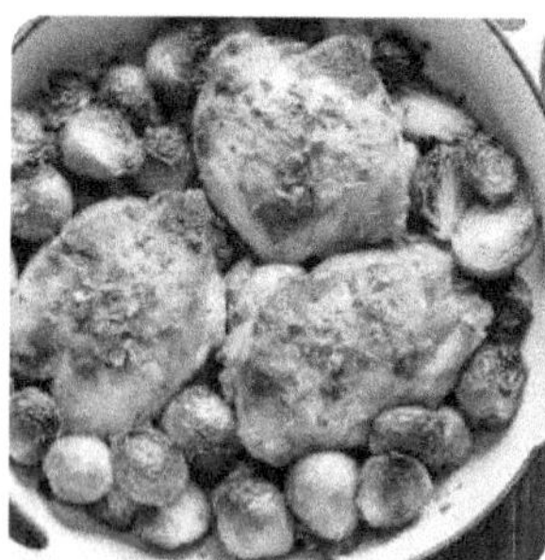

Ingredients

- 4 chicken thighs
- 1 lb Brussels sprouts, halved
- 2 tbsp olive oil
- 2 cloves garlic, minced
- Salt and pepper to taste

Directions

1. Preheat the oven to 400°F (200°C).
2. Place the chicken thighs and Brussels sprouts on a baking sheet.
3. Drizzle with olive oil and top with minced garlic.
4. Season with salt and pepper.
5. Bake for 25-30 minutes or until the chicken is cooked through and the Brussels sprouts are tender.
6. Serve immediately.

Ingredient Tips:

- Chicken Thighs: Higher in fat than chicken breasts but still provide high-quality protein.
- Brussels Sprouts: Low in calories and high in fiber, making them a great vegetable for blood sugar control.

Lentil and Vegetable Stew

A hearty and nutritious lentil and vegetable stew, perfect for a comforting and satisfying dinner.

Servings: 4 | Prep Time: 10 mins | Cook Time: 30 mins | Carbs per Serving: 30g

<table>
<tr><td colspan="2">NUTRIENT CONTENT (PER SERVING):</td></tr>
<tr><td>Calories: 220</td><td>Sugars: 8g</td></tr>
<tr><td>Total Fat: 5g</td><td>Fiber: 10g</td></tr>
<tr><td>Protein: 12g</td><td>Sodium: 350mg</td></tr>
<tr><td>Carbohydrates: 30g</td><td></td></tr>
</table>

Ingredients

- 1 cup lentils, rinsed
- 1 cup diced tomatoes
- 1 carrot, diced
- 1 zucchini, diced
- 1 onion, diced
- 2 cloves garlic, minced
- 4 cups vegetable broth (low sodium)
- 1 tbsp olive oil
- 1 tsp cumin
- 1 tsp paprika
- Salt and pepper to taste

Directions

1. In a large pot, heat the olive oil over medium heat.
2. Add the garlic and onion and sauté until softened.
3. Add the carrot and zucchini and cook for a few more minutes.
4. Stir in the cumin and paprika and cook for another minute.
5. Add the lentils, diced tomatoes, and vegetable broth.
6. Bring to a boil, then reduce the heat and simmer for 25-30 minutes, or until the lentils are tender.
7. Season with salt and pepper to taste and serve hot.

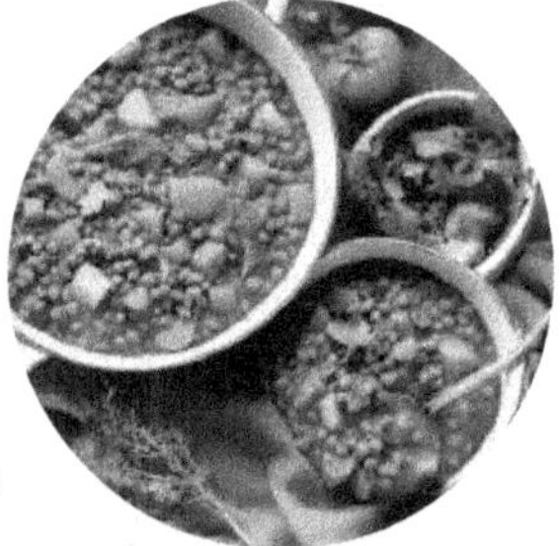

Ingredient Tips:

- Lentils: High in protein and fiber, helping to manage blood sugar levels.
- Vegetables: Adding a variety of vegetables increases the fiber content, which helps manage blood sugar levels.

Stuffed Bell Peppers with Ground Turkey

Tasty stuffed bell peppers filled with a seasoned ground turkey mixture, perfect for a hearty and balanced dinner.

NUTRIENT CONTENT (PER SERVING):
- Calories: 320
- Total Fat: 14g
- Protein: 25g
- Carbohydrates: 20g
- Sugars: 7g
- Fiber: 6g
- Sodium: 350mg

Servings: 4 | Prep Time: 15 mins | Cook Time:30 mins | Carbs per Serving :20g

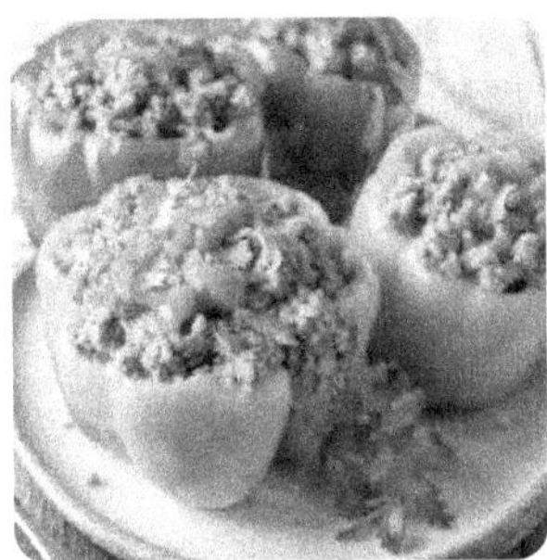

Ingredients

- 4 bell peppers
- 1 lb ground turkey
- 1 cup quinoa, cooked
- 1 cup diced tomatoes
- 1 onion, diced
- 2 cloves garlic, minced
- 1 tbsp olive oil
- 1 tsp cumin
- 1 tsp paprika
- Salt and pepper to taste

Directions

1. Preheat the oven to 375°F (190°C).
2. Cut the tops off the bell peppers and remove the seeds and membranes.
3. In a large skillet, heat the olive oil over medium heat.
4. Add the garlic and onion and sauté until softened.
5. Add the ground turkey and cook until browned.
6. Stir in the cooked quinoa, diced tomatoes, cumin, paprika, salt, and pepper.
7. Fill each bell pepper with the turkey mixture and place them in a baking dish.
8. Bake for 25-30 minutes or until the peppers are tender.

Ingredient Tips:

- Ground Turkey: Lean and high in protein, helping to keep you full and manage blood sugar levels.
- Quinoa: A high-protein grain that is also rich in fiber, helping to manage blood sugar levels.

Grilled Shrimp Tacos with Avocado

Flavorful grilled shrimp tacos topped with avocado and fresh veggies, perfect for a light and satisfying dinner.

NUTRIENT CONTENT (PER SERVING):
- Calories: 310
- Total Fat: 14g
- Protein: 25g
- Carbohydrates: 28g
- Sugars: 4g
- Fiber: 6g
- Sodium: 400mg

Servings: 4 | Prep Time: 15 mins | Cook Time: 6 mins | Carbs per Serving: 28g

Ingredients

- 1 lb shrimp, peeled and deveined
- 1 avocado, diced
- 1 cup shredded cabbage
- 1/4 cup red onion, diced
- 1/4 cup cilantro, chopped
- 8 small corn tortillas
- 2 tbsp olive oil
- 1 tbsp lime juice
- 1 tsp chili powder
- Salt and pepper to taste

Directions

1. In a bowl, combine the shrimp, olive oil, lime juice, chili powder, salt, and pepper.
2. Preheat the grill to medium-high heat.
3. Grill the shrimp for 2-3 minutes per side, or until cooked through.
4. Warm the corn tortillas on the grill.
5. Assemble the tacos by topping each tortilla with shrimp, avocado, shredded cabbage, red onion, and cilantro.

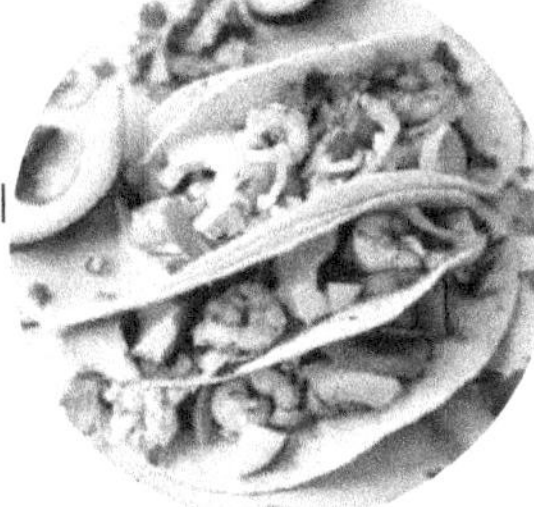

Ingredient Tips:

- Shrimp: Low in calories and high in protein, making them a great option for blood sugar control.
- Avocado: Provides healthy fats and fiber, aiding in blood sugar control.

Eggplant Parmesan

A healthier version of the classic eggplant Parmesan, perfect for a delicious and satisfying dinner.

Servings: 4 | Prep Time: 15 mins | Cook Time:30 mins | Carbs per Serving :20g

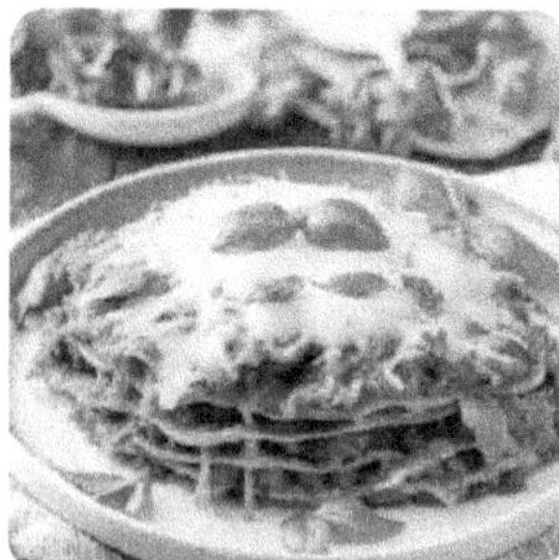

Ingredients

- 2 large eggplants, sliced
- 2 cups marinara sauce (low sodium)
- 1 cup mozzarella cheese, shredded
- 1/4 cup Parmesan cheese, grated
- 1/4 cup breadcrumbs (optional)
- 2 tbsp olive oil
- 2 cloves garlic, minced
- 1 tsp dried basil
- Salt and pepper to taste

Directions

1. Preheat the oven to 375°F (190°C).
2. Place the eggplant slices on a baking sheet and drizzle with olive oil.
3. Bake for 20 minutes, or until tender.
4. In a baking dish, spread a layer of marinara sauce.
5. Add a layer of eggplant slices, followed by a sprinkle of mozzarella cheese, Parmesan cheese, garlic, and basil.
6. Repeat the layers, ending with a layer of cheese on top.
7. Sprinkle breadcrumbs on top (if using).
8. Bake for 25-30 minutes, or until the cheese is melted and bubbly.

Ingredient Tips:

- Eggplant: Low in calories and high in fiber, making it a great vegetable for blood sugar control.
- Cheese: Provides protein and fat, helping to manage blood sugar levels.

Turkey & Spinach Stuffed Portobello Mushrooms

Savory turkey and spinach stuffed portobello mushrooms, perfect for a nutritious and filling dinner.

Servings: 4 | Prep Time: 15 mins | Cook Time:25 mins | Carbs per Serving: 8g

Ingredients

- 4 large portobello mushrooms, stems removed
- 1 lb ground turkey
- 2 cups fresh spinach, chopped
- 1/2 cup ricotta cheese
- 1/4 cup Parmesan cheese, grated
- 1 clove garlic, minced
- 1 tbsp olive oil
- Salt and pepper to taste

Directions

1. Preheat the oven to 375°F (190°C).
2. In a large skillet, heat the olive oil over medium heat.
3. Add the garlic and ground turkey and cook until browned.
4. Stir in the chopped spinach and cook until wilted.
5. Remove from heat and stir in the ricotta cheese, Parmesan cheese, salt, and pepper.
6. Stuff each portobello mushroom cap with the turkey mixture.
7. Place the stuffed mushrooms on a baking sheet and bake for 20-25 minutes, or until the mushrooms are tender.

Ingredient Tips:

- Portobello Mushrooms: Low in calories and high in fiber, making them a great vegetable for blood sugar control.
- Spinach: Provides vitamins and minerals, enhancing the nutritional profile of the dish.

Lemon Herb Grilled Chicken

Tender and flavorful lemon herb grilled chicken, perfect for a simple and healthy dinner.

Servings: 4 | Prep Time: 10 mins | Cook Time:14 mins | Carbs per Serving :2g

NUTRIENT CONTENT (PER SERVING):

- Calories: 240
- Total Fat: 12g
- Protein: 28g
- Carbohydrates: 2g
- Sugars: 0g
- Fiber: 0g
- Sodium: 200mg

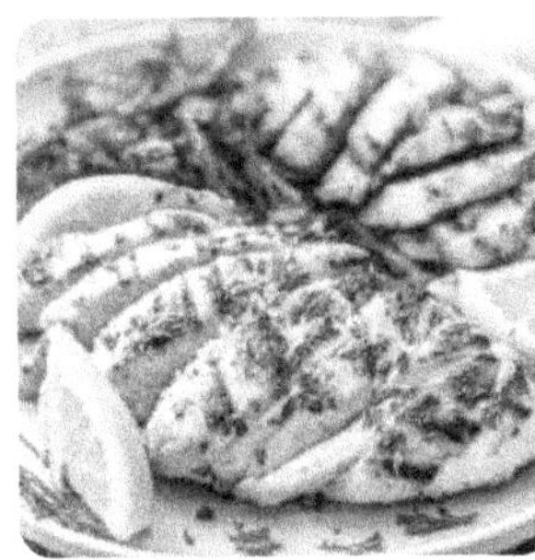

Ingredients

- 4 chicken breasts
- 2 tbsp olive oil
- 2 tbsp lemon juice
- 2 cloves garlic, minced
- 1 tsp dried oregano
- 1 tsp dried thyme
- Salt and pepper to taste

Directions

1. In a bowl, combine the olive oil, lemon juice, garlic, oregano, thyme, salt, and pepper.
2. Add the chicken breasts and marinate for at least 30 minutes.
3. Preheat the grill to medium-high heat.
4. Grill the chicken for 5-7 minutes per side, or until cooked through.
5. Serve immediately.

Ingredient Tips:

- Chicken Breast: Lean and high in protein, helping to keep you full and manage blood sugar levels.
- Lemon: Adds flavor without adding extra calories or sugar.

Spaghetti Squash with Tomato & Basil

A light and flavorful spaghetti squash dish with fresh tomatoes and basil, perfect for a low-carb and delicious dinner.

NUTRIENT CONTENT (PER SERVING):

- Calories: 180
- Total Fat: 10g
- Protein: 3g
- Carbohydrates: 15g
- Sugars: 6g
- Fiber: 4g
- Sodium: 100mg

Servings: 4 | Prep Time: 10 mins | Cook Time:40 mins | Carbs per Serving: 1g

Ingredients

- 1 large spaghetti squash
- 2 cups cherry tomatoes, halved
- 1/4 cup fresh basil, chopped
- 2 tbsp olive oil
- 2 cloves garlic, minced
- Salt and pepper to taste

Directions

1. Preheat the oven to 375°F (190°C).
2. Cut the spaghetti squash in half lengthwise and remove the seeds.
3. Place the squash halves cut side down on a baking sheet and bake for 30-40 minutes, or until tender.
4. Using a fork, scrape out the spaghetti-like strands from the squash.
5. In a large skillet, heat the olive oil over medium heat.
6. Add the garlic and sauté until fragrant.
7. Add the cherry tomatoes and cook until softened.
8. Stir in the spaghetti squash strands and fresh basil.
9. Season with salt and pepper to taste and serve hot.

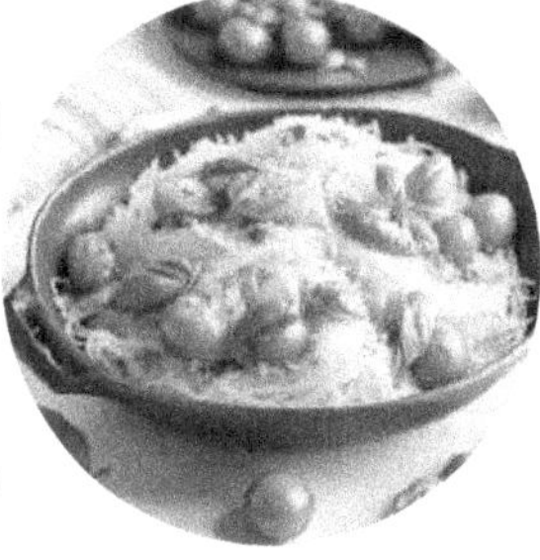

Ingredient Tips:

- Spaghetti Squash: A low-carb alternative to pasta, high in fiber and vitamins.
- Cherry Tomatoes: Low in calories and high in vitamins, adding flavor and nutrition.

Salmon with Asparagus and Lemon

A simple and delicious salmon dish served with roasted asparagus and a hint of lemon, perfect for a nutritious and balanced dinner.

Servings: 4 | Prep Time: 10 mins | Cook Time:20 mins | Carbs per Serving :8g

NUTRIENT CONTENT (PER SERVING):
• Calories: 300   • Sugars: 2g • Total Fat: 18g   • Fiber: 4g • Protein: 25g • Carbohydrates: 8g   • Sodium: 150mg

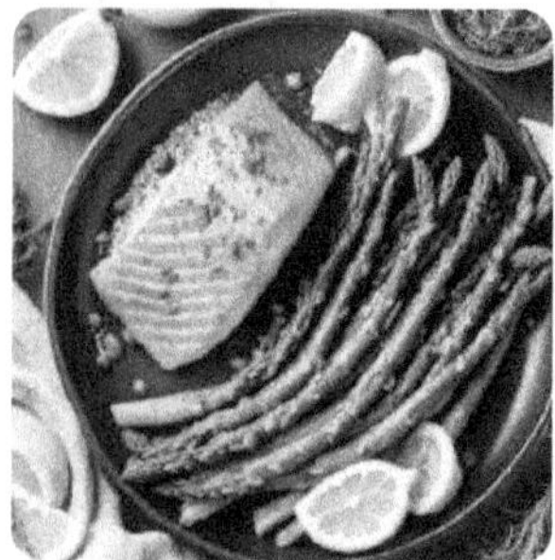

Ingredients

- 4 salmon fillets
- 1 lb asparagus, trimmed
- 2 tbsp olive oil
- 2 tbsp lemon juice
- 2 cloves garlic, minced
- Salt and pepper to taste

Directions

1. Preheat the oven to 400°F (200°C).
2. Place the salmon fillets and asparagus on a baking sheet.
3. Drizzle with olive oil and lemon juice, and top with minced garlic.
4. Season with salt and pepper.
5. Bake for 15-20 minutes, or until the salmon is cooked through and the asparagus is tender.
6. Serve immediately.

Ingredient Tips:

- Salmon: High in omega-3 fatty acids, which are beneficial for heart health and blood sugar control.
- Asparagus: Low in calories and high in fiber, making it a great vegetable for blood sugar control.

Chicken and Broccoli Stir-Fry

A quick and easy chicken and broccoli stir-fry, perfect for a healthy and balanced dinner.

Servings: 4 | Prep Time: 10 mins | Cook Time:15 mins | Carbs per Serving: 10g

NUTRIENT CONTENT (PER SERVING):
• Calories: 250   • Sugars: 4g • Total Fat: 14g   • Fiber: 4g • Protein: 25g • Carbohydrates: 10g   • Sodium: 400mg

Ingredients

- 1 lb chicken breast, sliced thin
- 3 cups broccoli florets
- 1 bell pepper, sliced
- 1 onion, sliced
- 2 tbsp soy sauce (low sodium)
- 1 tbsp sesame oil
- 1 tbsp olive oil
- 2 cloves garlic, minced
- 1 tsp ginger, minced
- Salt and pepper to taste

Directions

1. In a large skillet, heat the olive oil over medium-high heat.
2. Add the garlic and ginger and sauté until fragrant.
3. Add the chicken and cook until browned.
4. Add the broccoli, bell pepper, and onion and cook until tender-crisp.
5. Stir in the soy sauce and sesame oil.
6. Season with salt and pepper to taste and serve hot.

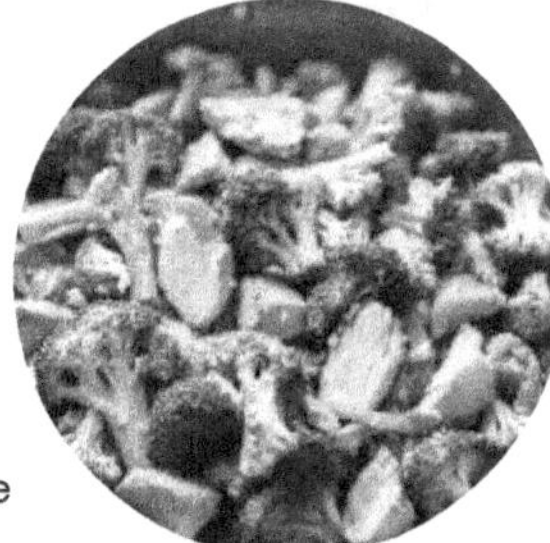

Ingredient Tips:

- Chicken Breast: Lean and high in protein, helping to keep you full and manage blood sugar levels.
- Broccoli: Low in calories and high in fiber, making it a great vegetable for blood sugar control.

Quinoa & Black Bean Stuffed Zucchini

Tasty quinoa and black bean stuffed zucchini boats, perfect for a nutritious and filling dinner.

Servings: 4 | Prep Time: 15 mins | Cook Time:25 mins | Carbs per Serving :22g

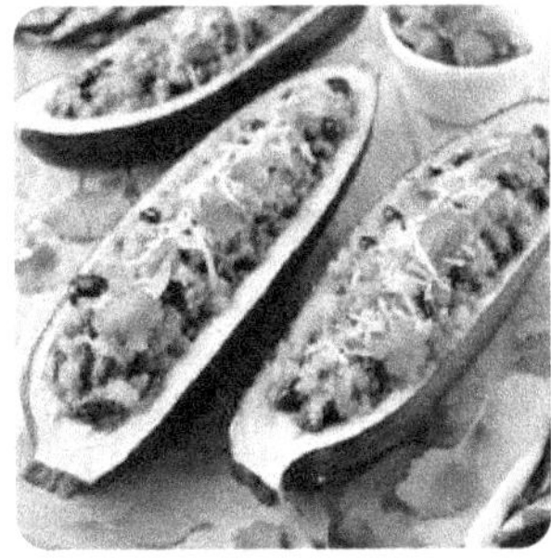

Ingredients

- 4 large zucchinis, halved lengthwise and seeds removed
- 1 cup cooked quinoa
- 1 cup black beans, rinsed and drained
- 1 cup diced tomatoes
- 1/4 cup red onion, diced
- 1/4 cup cilantro, chopped
- 1 tbsp olive oil
- 1 tsp cumin
- Salt and pepper to taste

Directions

1. Preheat the oven to 375°F (190°C).
2. In a large bowl, combine the cooked quinoa, black beans, diced tomatoes, red onion, cilantro, olive oil, cumin, salt, and pepper.
3. Stuff each zucchini half with the quinoa mixture and place them on a baking sheet.
4. Bake for 20-25 minutes, or until the zucchinis are tender.
5. Serve immediately.

Ingredient Tips:

- Quinoa: A high-protein grain that is also rich in fiber, helping to manage blood sugar levels.
- Black Beans: High in protein and fiber, helping to manage blood sugar levels.

Baked Cod with Tomatoes & Olives

A delicious baked cod dish with tomatoes and olives, perfect for a light and flavorful dinner.

Servings: 4 | Prep Time: 10 mins | Cook Time:25 mins | Carbs per Serving: 5g

Ingredients

- 4 cod fillets
- 2 cups cherry tomatoes, halved
- 1/4 cup black olives, sliced
- 2 cloves garlic, minced
- 2 tbsp olive oil
- 1 tbsp lemon juice
- 1 tsp dried oregano
- Salt and pepper to taste

Directions

1. Preheat the oven to 375°F (190°C).
2. Place the cod fillets in a baking dish.
3. In a bowl, combine the cherry tomatoes, black olives, garlic, olive oil, lemon juice, oregano, salt, and pepper.
4. Spoon the tomato mixture over the cod fillets.
5. Bake for 20-25 minutes, or until the cod is cooked through.
6. Serve immediately.

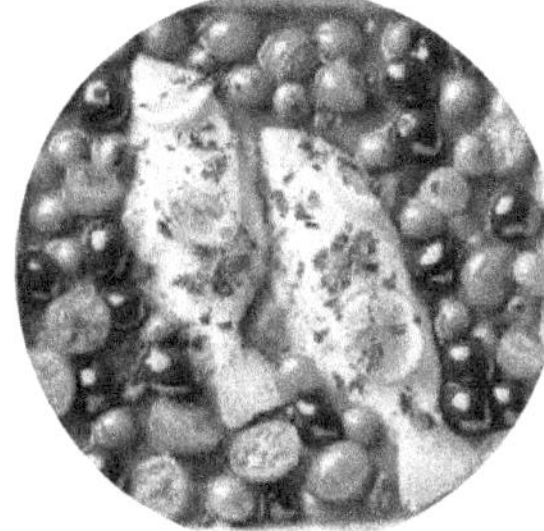

Ingredient Tips:

- Cod: A lean and high-protein fish, making it a great option for blood sugar control.
- Tomatoes: Low in calories and high in vitamins, adding flavor and nutrition.

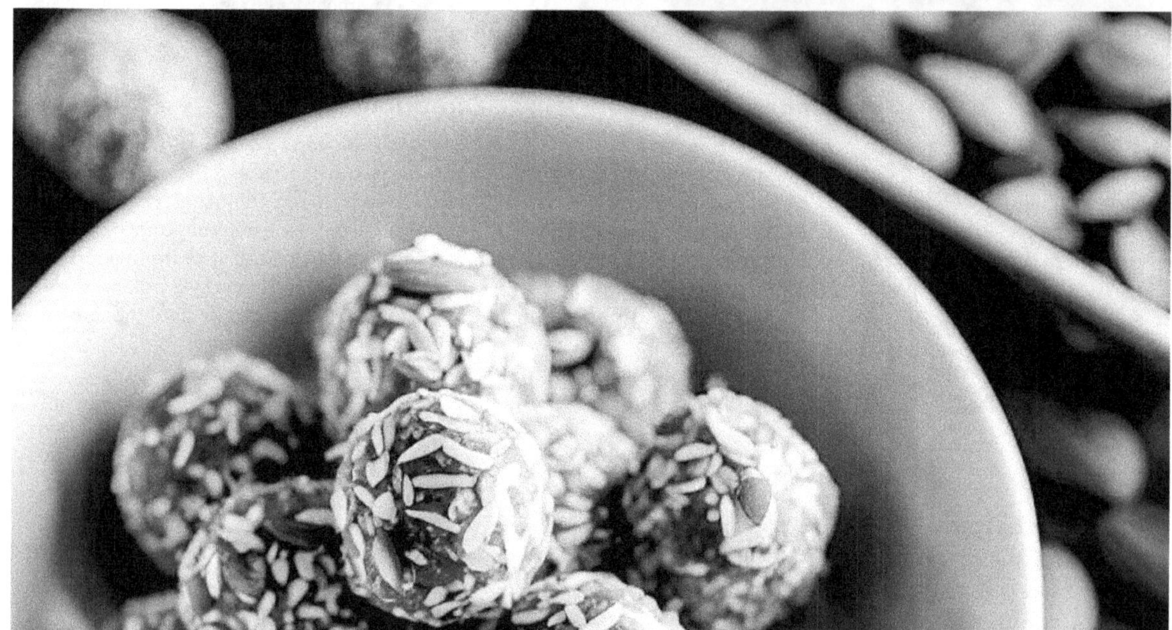

Chapter Eight

Desserts Recipes

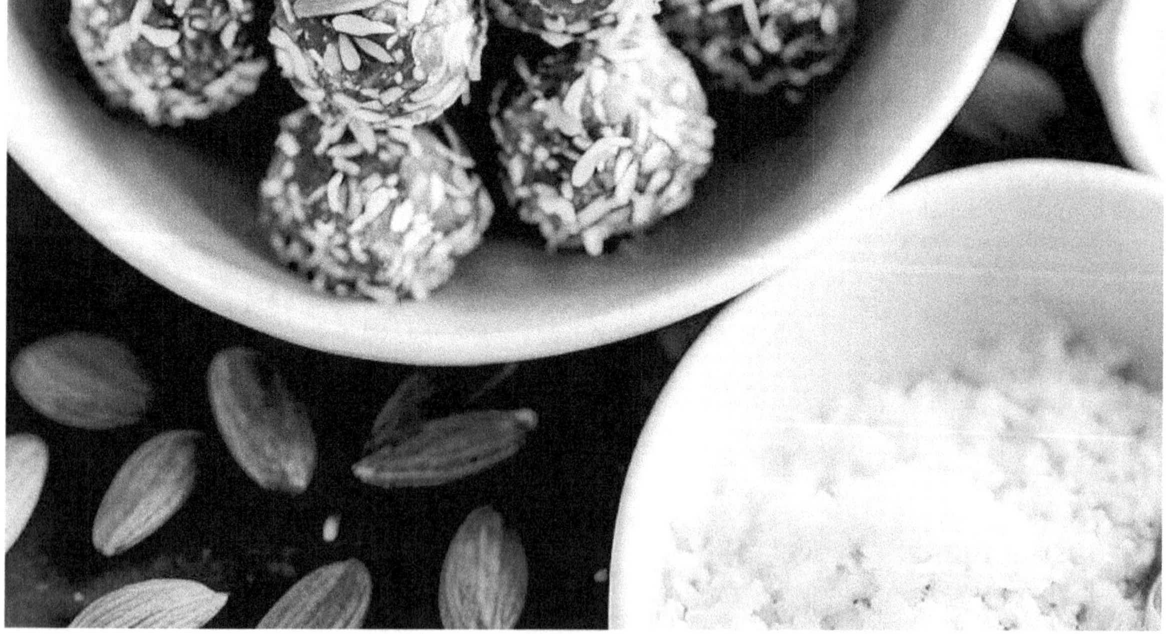

Avocado Chocolate Mousse

A creamy and delicious chocolate mousse made with avocado for a healthy twist.

Servings: 4 | Prep Time: 10 mins | Cook Time:0 mins | Carbs per Serving :12g

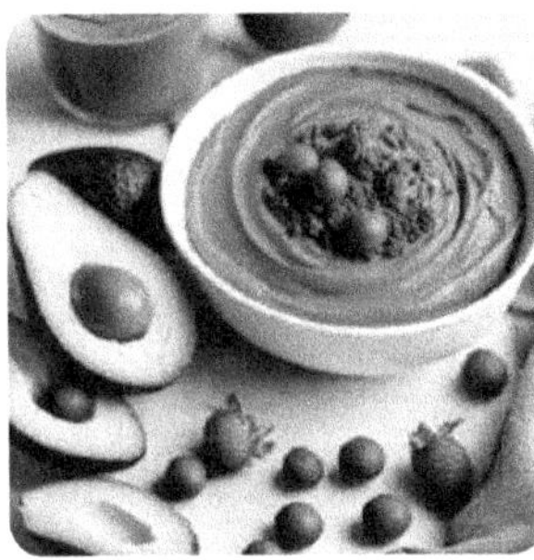

Ingredients

- 2 ripe avocados
- 1/4 cup unsweetened cocoa powder
- 1/4 cup unsweetened almond milk
- 2 tbsp stevia or other preferred sweetener
- 1 tsp vanilla extract
- Fresh berries for garnish

Directions

1. Cut the avocados in half, remove the pit, and scoop the flesh into a blender.
2. Add the cocoa powder, almond milk, stevia, and vanilla extract.
3. Blend until smooth and creamy.
4. Divide into serving bowls and chill for at least 30 minutes.
5. Garnish with fresh berries before serving.

Ingredient Tips:

-
- Avocado: Provides healthy fats and fiber, aiding in blood sugar control.
- Cocoa Powder: Rich in antioxidants and adds a deep chocolate flavor without added sugars.

Chia Seed Pudding

: A simple and nutritious chia seed pudding that's perfect for a healthy dessert.

Servings: 2 | Prep Time: 5 mins | Cook Time:0 mins | Carbs per Serving: 10g

Ingredients

- 1/4 cup chia seeds
- 1 cup unsweetened almond milk
- 1 tsp vanilla extract
- 1 tbsp stevia or other preferred sweetener
- Fresh berries for topping

Directions

1. In a bowl, combine chia seeds, almond milk, vanilla extract, and sweetener.
2. Stir well and let sit for 5 minutes, then stir again to prevent clumping.
3. Cover and refrigerate for at least 4 hours or overnight.
4. Serve chilled, topped with fresh berries.

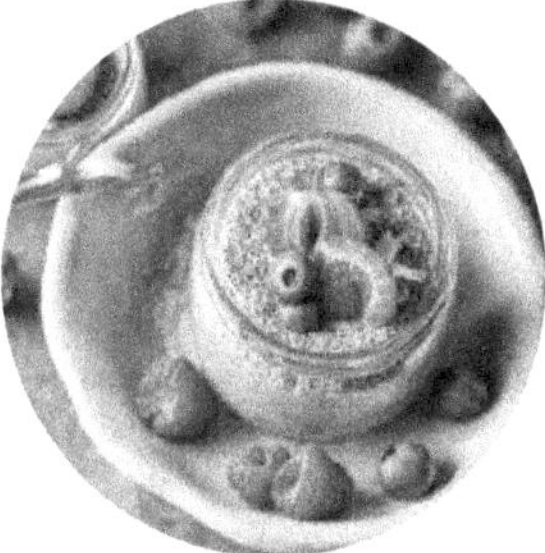

Ingredient Tips:

- Chia Seeds: High in fiber and omega-3 fatty acids, helping to manage blood sugar levels.
- Almond Milk: Low in carbohydrates and calories, making it a great base for puddings.

Greek Yogurt Parfait

A delicious and protein-packed Greek yogurt parfait layered with fresh fruit and nuts.

Servings: 5 | Prep Time: 5 mins | Cook Time:0 mins | Carbs per Serving :20g

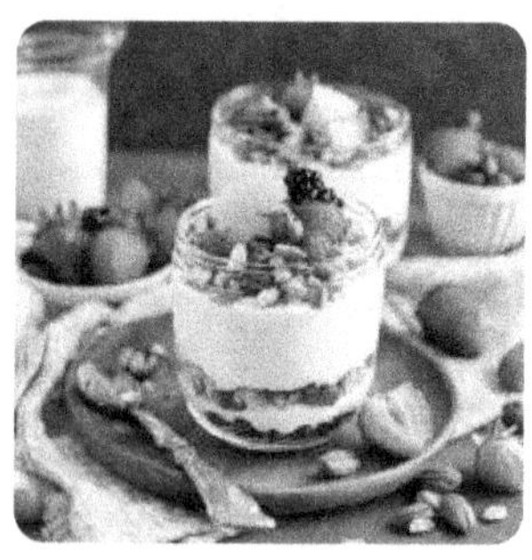

Ingredients

- 1 cup plain Greek yogurt
- 1/2 cup mixed berries (blueberries, strawberries, raspberries)
- 1/4 cup granola (low sugar)
- 1 tbsp chopped nuts (almonds or walnuts)

Directions

1. In a glass or bowl, layer Greek yogurt, berries, granola, and nuts.
2. Repeat the layers until all ingredients are used.
3. Serve immediately or refrigerate until ready to eat.

Ingredient Tips:

- Greek Yogurt: High in protein and low in carbohydrates, helping to keep blood sugar levels stable.
- Berries: Low glycemic index fruits that are rich in antioxidants and fiber.

Almond Flour Cookies

Soft and chewy cookies made with almond flour, perfect for a low-carb dessert.

Servings: 12 | Prep Time: 10 mins | Cook Time :12mins | Carbs per Serving: 5g

Ingredients

- 2 cups almond flour
- 1/4 cup coconut oil, melted
- 1/4 cup stevia or other preferred sweetener
- 1 tsp vanilla extract
- 1/4 tsp baking soda
- A pinch of salt
- 1 egg

Directions

1. Preheat the oven to 350°F (175°C).
2. In a bowl, combine almond flour, baking soda, and salt.
3. In another bowl, mix melted coconut oil, stevia, vanilla extract, and egg.
4. Combine the wet and dry ingredients and mix until a dough forms.
5. Scoop spoonfuls of dough onto a baking sheet lined with parchment paper.
6. Flatten the dough slightly with a fork.
7. Bake for 10-12 minutes or until golden brown.
8. Let cool on a wire rack before serving.

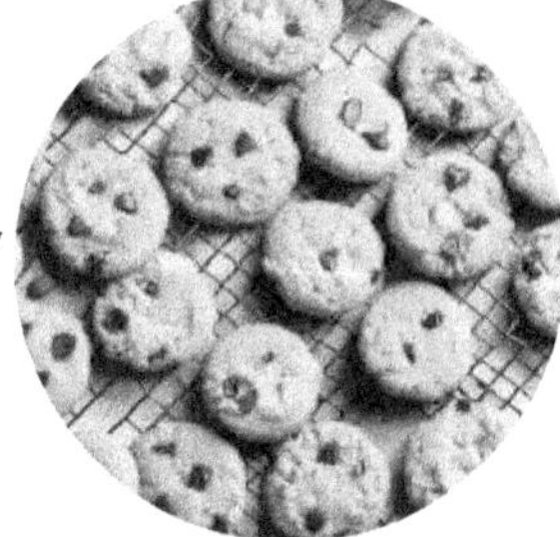

Ingredient Tips:

- Almond Flour: Low in carbohydrates and high in healthy fats and protein, making it suitable for managing blood sugar levels.
- Coconut Oil: Provides healthy fats and a delicious flavor to the cookies.

Berry and Spinach Smoothie

A refreshing and nutritious smoothie with berries and spinach, perfect for a light dessert.

Servings: 2 | Prep Time: 5 mins | Cook Time:0 mins | Carbs per Serving :15g

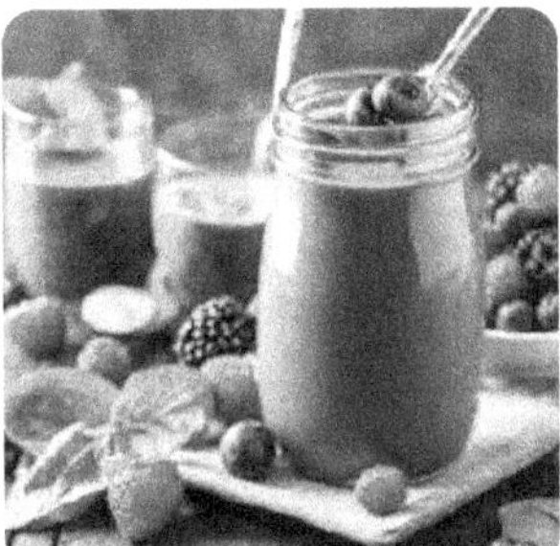

Ingredients

- 1 cup mixed berries (strawberries, blueberries, raspberries)
- 1 handful of fresh spinach
- 1/2 cup unsweetened almond milk
- 1/2 cup plain Greek yogurt
- 1 tbsp chia seeds
- 1 tbsp stevia or other preferred sweetener

Directions

1. In a blender, combine all ingredients and blend until smooth.
2. Pour into glasses and serve immediately.

Ingredient Tips:

- Berries: Low glycemic index fruits that help manage blood sugar levels.
- Spinach: Adds fiber and essential nutrients without altering the flavor of the smoothie.

Coconut and Almond Energy Balls

Easy-to-make energy balls with coconut and almonds, perfect for a quick and healthy dessert.

Servings: 12 | Prep Time: 10 mins | Cook Time :0 mins | Carbs per Serving: 6g

Ingredients

- 1 cup almond flour
- 1/2 cup shredded unsweetened coconut
- 1/4 cup coconut oil, melted
- 2 tbsp chia seeds
- 2 tbsp stevia or other preferred sweetener
- 1 tsp vanilla extract

Directions

1. In a bowl, combine all ingredients and mix until well combined.
2. Roll the mixture into small balls and place on a baking sheet lined with parchment paper.
3. Refrigerate for at least 30 minutes before serving.

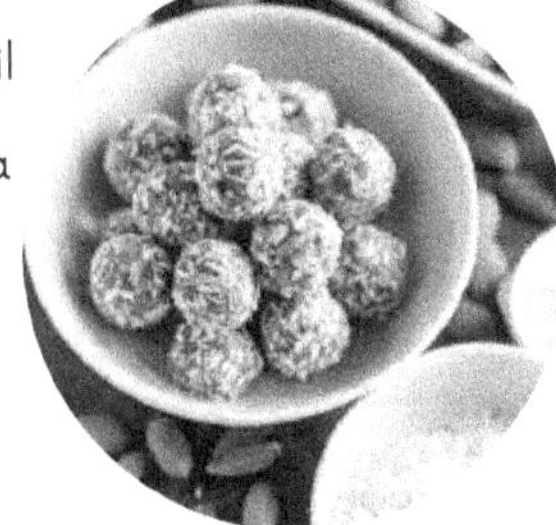

Ingredient Tips:

- Almond Flour: Low in carbohydrates and high in healthy fats and protein.
- Chia Seeds: High in fiber and omega-3 fatty acids, helping to manage blood sugar levels.

Blueberry Almond Crisp

A delightful blueberry almond crisp that's both nutritious and satisfying.

Servings: 4 | Prep Time: 10 mins | Cook Time:30 mins | Carbs per Serving :15g

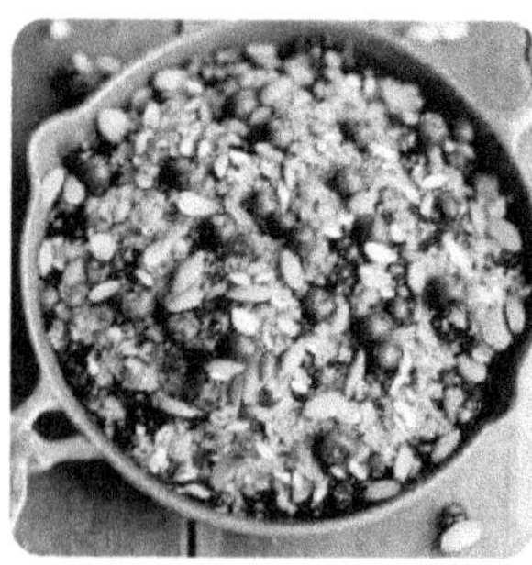

Ingredients

- 2 cups fresh blueberries
- 1/2 cup almond flour
- 1/4 cup chopped almonds
- 2 tbsp coconut oil, melted
- 1 tbsp stevia or other preferred sweetener
- 1 tsp vanilla extract

Directions

1. Preheat the oven to 350°F (175°C).
2. Place the blueberries in a baking dish.
3. In a bowl, combine almond flour, chopped almonds, melted coconut oil, stevia, and vanilla extract.
4. Sprinkle the almond mixture over the blueberries.
5. Bake for 25-30 minutes, until the topping is golden brown.
6. Serve warm.

Ingredient Tips:

- Berries: Low glycemic index fruits that help manage blood sugar levels.
- Spinach: Adds fiber and essential nutrients without altering the flavor of the smoothie.

Coconut and Almond Energy Balls

Easy-to-make energy balls with coconut and almonds, perfect for a quick and healthy dessert.

Servings: 12 | Prep Time: 10 mins | Cook Time :0 mins | Carbs per Serving: 6g

Ingredients

- 1 cup almond flour
- 1/2 cup shredded unsweetened coconut
- 1/4 cup coconut oil, melted
- 2 tbsp chia seeds
- 2 tbsp stevia or other preferred sweetener
- 1 tsp vanilla extract

Directions

1. In a bowl, combine all ingredients and mix until well combined.
2. Roll the mixture into small balls and place on a baking sheet lined with parchment paper.
3. Refrigerate for at least 30 minutes before serving.

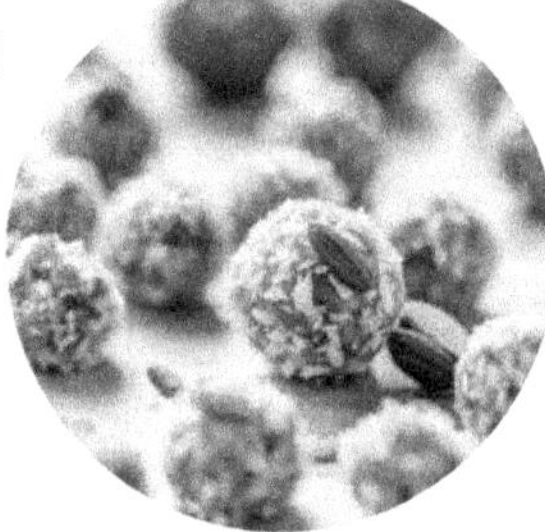

Ingredient Tips:

- Almond Flour: Low in carbohydrates and high in healthy fats and protein.
- Chia Seeds: High in fiber and omega-3 fatty acids, helping to manage blood sugar levels.

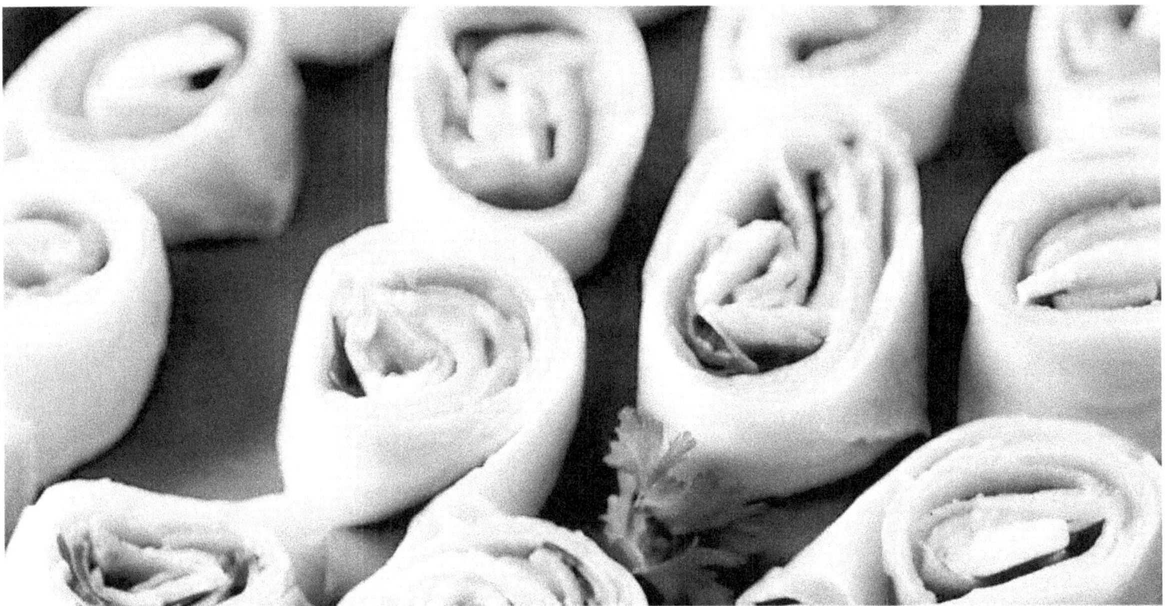

Chapter Nine

Snacks and Appetizers Recipes

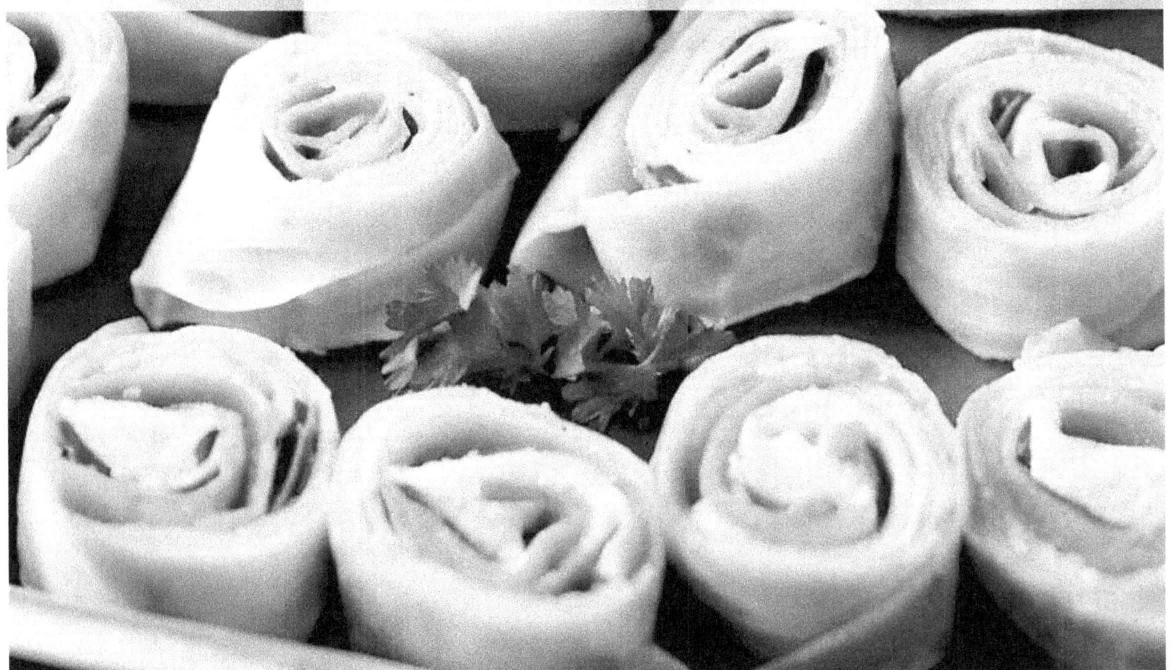

Apple and Walnut Salad

A simple and refreshing apple and walnut salad with a dressing.

Servings: 2 | Prep Time: 5 mins | Cook Time:0 mins | Carbs per Serving :15g

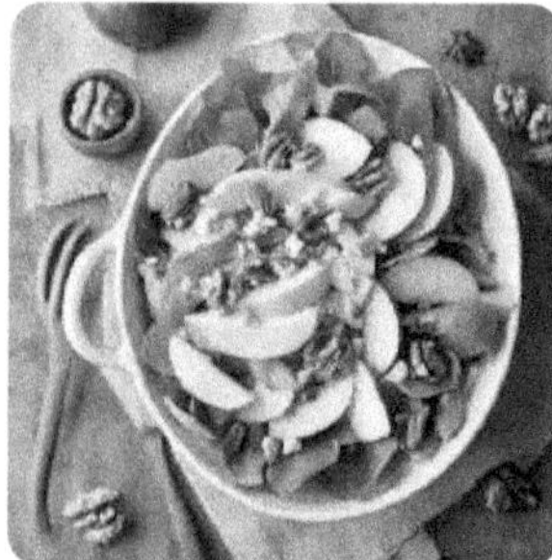

Ingredients

- 2 medium apples, thinly sliced
- 1/4 cup chopped walnuts
- 4 cups mixed greens
- 2 tbsp olive oil
- 1 tbsp apple cider vinegar
- Salt and pepper to taste

Directions

1. In a large bowl, combine the apples, walnuts, and mixed greens.
2. In a small bowl, whisk together the olive oil, apple cider vinegar, salt, and pepper.
3. Drizzle the dressing over the salad and toss to combine.
4. Serve immediately.

Ingredient Tips:

- Apples: Contain fiber and natural sweetness without a high glycemic index.
- Walnuts: Provide healthy fats and protein, aiding in blood sugar control.

Baked Pears with Cinnamon

Warm and spiced baked pears, a healthy and delicious dessert.

Servings: 4 | Prep Time: 5 mins | Cook Time 25 mins | Carbs per Serving: 20g

Ingredients

- 2 ripe pears, halved and cored
- 1 tsp cinnamon
- 1 tbsp chopped walnuts
- 1 tbsp melted coconut oil
- 1 tbsp stevia or other preferred sweetener

Directions

1. Preheat the oven to 350°F (175°C).
2. Place the pear halves in a baking dish.
3. Sprinkle with cinnamon and chopped walnuts.
4. Drizzle with melted coconut oil and stevia.
5. Bake for 20-25 minutes, until the pears are tender.
6. Serve warm.

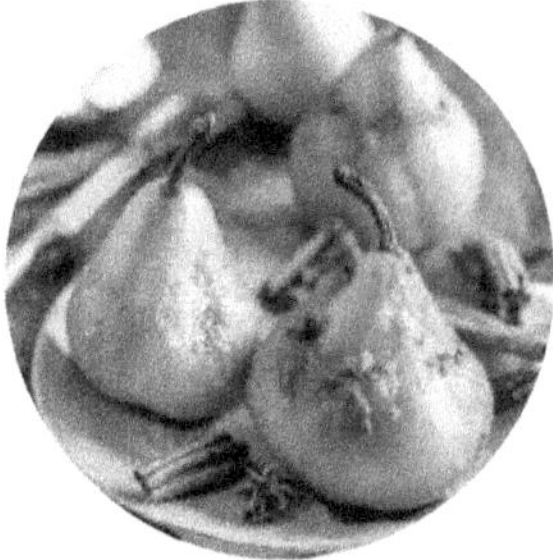

Ingredient Tips:

- Blueberries: Low glycemic index fruits that help manage blood sugar levels.
- Almond Flour: Provides healthy fats and protein, aiding in blood sugar control.

Blueberry Almond Crisp

NUTRIENT CONTENT (PER SERVING):

- Calories: 140
- Total Fat: 9g
- Protein: 3g
- Carbohydrates: 15g
- Sugars: 7g
- Fiber: 5g
- Sodium: 0mg

: A delightful blueberry almond crisp that's both nutritious and satisfying.

Servings: 4 | Prep Time: 10 mins | Cook Time:0 3mins | Carbs per Serving :15g

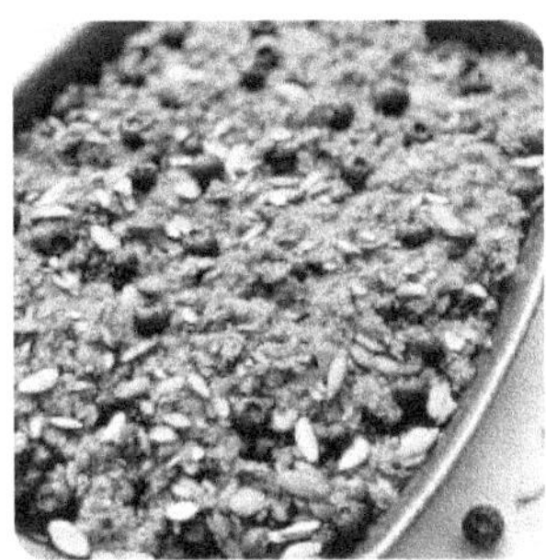

Ingredients

- 2 cups fresh blueberries
- 1/2 cup almond flour
- 1/4 cup chopped almonds
- 2 tbsp coconut oil, melted
- 1 tbsp stevia or other preferred sweetener
- 1 tsp vanilla extract

Directions

1. Preheat the oven to 350°F (175°C).
2. Place the blueberries in a baking dish.
3. In a bowl, combine almond flour, chopped almonds, melted coconut oil, stevia, and vanilla extract.
4. Sprinkle the almond mixture over the blueberries.
5. Bake for 25-30 minutes, until the topping is golden brown.
6. Serve warm.

Ingredient Tips:

- Blueberries: Low glycemic index fruits that help manage blood sugar levels.
- Almond Flour: Provides healthy fats and protein, aiding in blood sugar control.

Pumpkin Protein Bars

NUTRIENT CONTENT (PER SERVING):

- Calories: 90
- Total Fat: 4g
- Protein: 6g
- Carbohydrates: 10g
- Sugars: 2g
- Fiber: 3g
- Sodium: 60mg

Healthy and protein-packed pumpkin bars, perfect for a fall-inspired dessert.

Servings: 8 | Prep Time: 10mins | Cook Time 25 mins | Carbs per Serving: 10g

Ingredients

- 1 cup canned pumpkin
- 1/2 cup almond flour
- 1/4 cup protein powder (vanilla or unflavored)
- 1/4 cup stevia or other preferred sweetener
- 1 tsp pumpkin pie spice
- 1 tsp vanilla extract
- 2 eggs

Directions

1. Preheat the oven to 350°F (175°C).
2. In a bowl, combine pumpkin, almond flour, protein powder, stevia, pumpkin pie spice, vanilla extract, and eggs.
3. Mix until well combined.
4. Pour the batter into a baking dish lined with parchment paper.
5. Bake for 20-25 minutes, until set and slightly golden.
6. Let cool before cutting into bars.

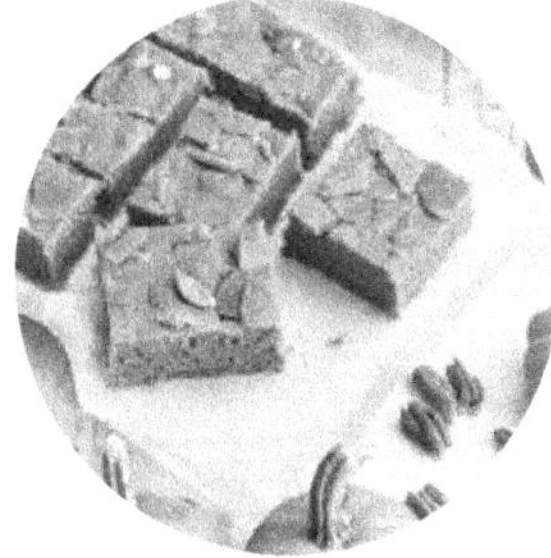

Ingredient Tips:

- Pumpkin: Low in calories and high in fiber, making it a great addition to desserts for blood sugar control.
- Protein Powder: Adds protein to help maintain steady blood sugar levels.

Avocado Deviled Eggs

A creamy and delicious twist on classic deviled eggs with healthy fats from avocado, perfect for a satisfying snack or appetizer.

Servings: 6 | Prep Time: 10 mins | Cook Time:0 0 mins | Carbs per Serving :2 g

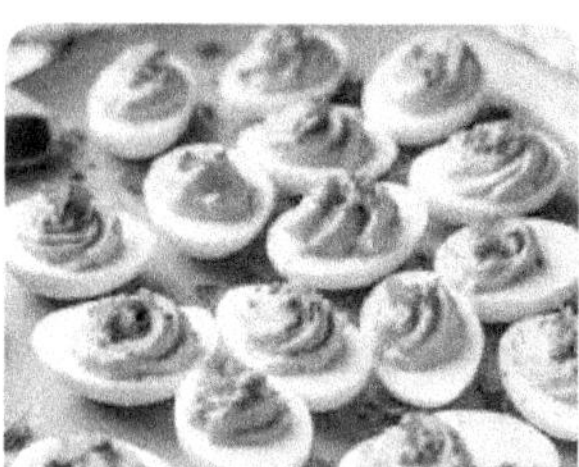

Ingredients

- 6 hard-boiled eggs
- 1 ripe avocado
- 1 tbsp lemon juice
- 1 tsp Dijon mustard
- Salt and pepper to taste
- Paprika for garnish

Directions

1. Peel the hard-boiled eggs and cut them in half lengthwise. Remove the yolks and place them in a bowl.
2. Mash the egg yolks with the avocado, lemon juice, and Dijon mustard until smooth.
3. Season with salt and pepper to taste.
4. Spoon the avocado mixture back into the egg whites.
5. Sprinkle with paprika and serve.

Ingredient Tips:

- Avocado: Provides healthy fats and fiber, aiding in blood sugar control.
- Eggs: A great source of protein that helps keep you full and manage blood sugar levels.

Cucumber and Hummus Bites

Refreshing cucumber slices topped with creamy hummus, perfect for a light and healthy snack.

Servings: 4   Prep Time: 10mins | Cook Time 0 mins | Carbs per Serving: 10g

Ingredients

- 1 cucumber, sliced into rounds
- 1 cup hummus
- 1 tbsp olive oil
- Paprika for garnish

Directions

1. Arrange the cucumber slices on a serving platter.
2. Top each slice with a dollop of hummus.
3. Drizzle with olive oil and sprinkle with paprika.
4. Serve immediately.

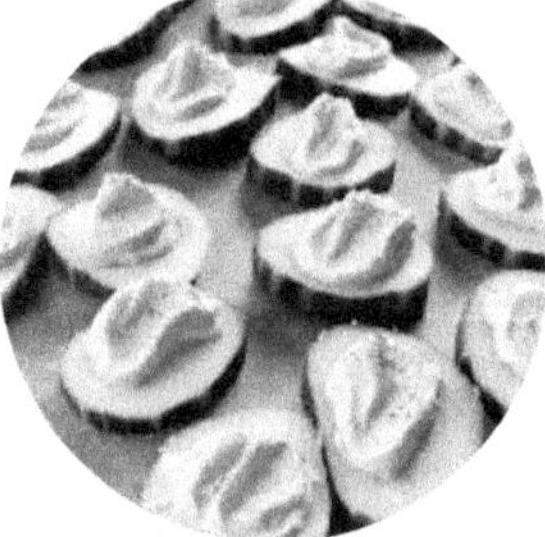

Ingredient Tips:

- Cucumber: Low in calories and high in water content, making it a refreshing and hydrating choice.
- Hummus: Provides protein and healthy fats, aiding in blood sugar control.

Greek Yogurt and Veggie Dip

A creamy Greek yogurt dip with fresh vegetables, perfect for a protein-packed snack.

Servings: 4 | Prep Time: 10 mins | Cook Time:0 0 mins | Carbs per Serving :4g

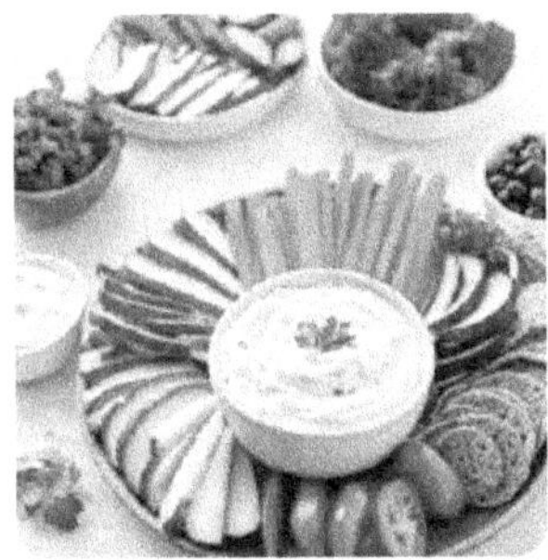

Ingredients

- 1 cup plain Greek yogurt
- 1 clove garlic, minced
- 1 tbsp lemon juice
- 1 tbsp fresh dill, chopped
- Salt and pepper to taste
- Assorted fresh vegetables (carrot sticks, bell pepper strips, cherry tomatoes)

Directions

1. In a bowl, combine the Greek yogurt, garlic, lemon juice, and dill.
2. Season with salt and pepper to taste.
3. Serve with assorted fresh vegetables for dipping.

Ingredient Tips:

- Greek Yogurt: High in protein and probiotics, which can help manage blood sugar levels.
- Fresh Vegetables: Provide fiber and essential nutrients, aiding in blood sugar control.

Turkey and Cheese Roll-Ups

Simple and tasty turkey and cheese roll-ups, perfect for a quick and satisfying snack.

Servings: 4 | Prep Time: 5mins | Cook Time 0 mins | Carbs per Serving: 1g

Ingredients

- 8 slices turkey breast
- 4 slices cheddar cheese
- 1 tbsp Dijon mustard

Directions

1. Spread a thin layer of Dijon mustard on each slice of turkey.
2. Place a slice of cheddar cheese on top of each turkey slice.
3. Roll up the turkey and cheese and secure with a toothpick if needed.
4. Serve immediately.

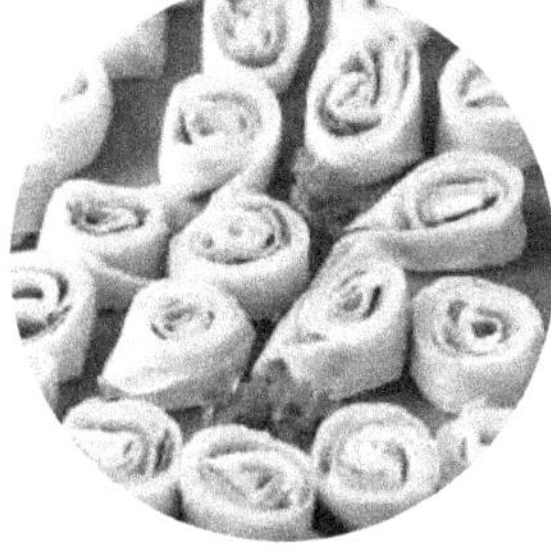

Ingredient Tips:

- Turkey Breast: Lean and high in protein, helping to keep you full and manage blood sugar levels.
- Cheddar Cheese: Provides protein and healthy fats, aiding in blood sugar control.

Spiced Nuts

A flavorful and crunchy mix of spiced nuts, perfect for a protein-packed snack.

Servings: 4 | Prep Time: 5 mins | Cook Time: 12 mins | Carbs per Serving :8g

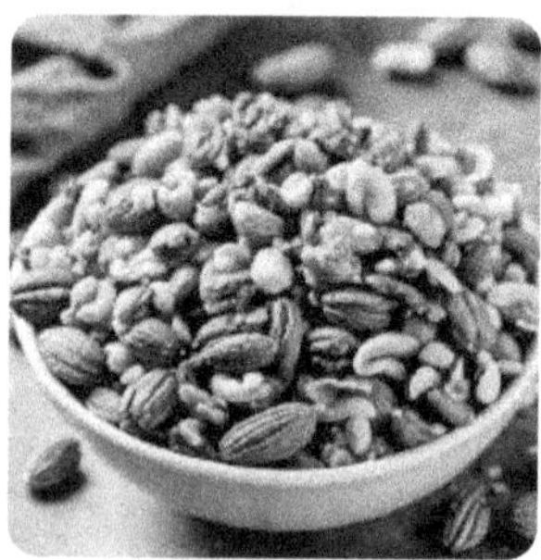

Ingredients

- 1 cup mixed nuts (almonds, cashews, walnuts)
- 1 tbsp olive oil
- 1 tsp chili powder
- 1/2 tsp cumin
- 1/2 tsp paprika
- Salt to taste

Directions

1. Preheat the oven to 350°F (175°C).
2. In a bowl, combine the mixed nuts, olive oil, chili powder, cumin, paprika, and salt.
3. Spread the nuts on a baking sheet in a single layer.
4. Bake for 10-12 minutes, stirring halfway through, until the nuts are toasted and fragrant.
5. Let cool before serving.

Ingredient Tips:

- Mixed Nuts: Provide healthy fats and protein, aiding in blood sugar control.
- Spices: Add flavor without extra calories or sugars.

Lentil and Veggie Lettuce Wraps

Tasty and nutritious lentil and veggie lettuce wraps, perfect for a light and healthy snack.

Servings: 4   Prep Time: 10mins | Cook Time 0 mins | Carbs per Serving: 14g

Ingredients

- 1 cup cooked lentils
- 1 carrot, shredded
- 1 bell pepper, diced
- 2 tbsp olive oil
- 1 tbsp soy sauce (low sodium)
- 1 tsp sesame oil
- 8 large lettuce leaves

Directions

1. In a bowl, combine the cooked lentils, shredded carrot, and diced bell pepper.
2. In a small bowl, whisk together the olive oil, soy sauce, and sesame oil.
3. Pour the dressing over the lentil and veggie mixture and toss to combine.
4. Spoon the lentil mixture onto the lettuce leaves.
5. Serve immediately.

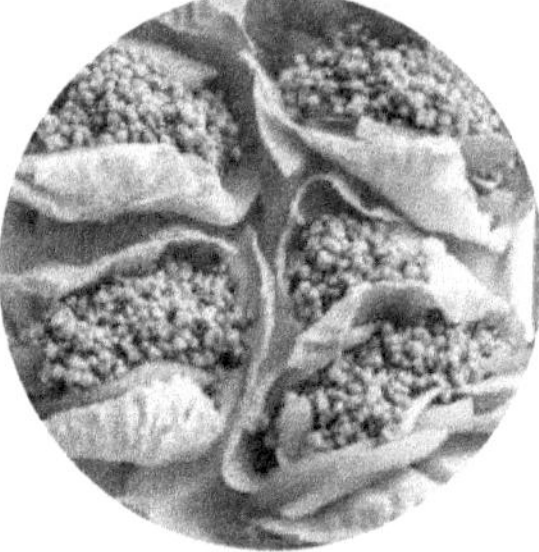

Ingredient Tips:

- Lentils: High in fiber and protein, helping to manage blood sugar levels.
- Lettuce: Low in calories and carbohydrates, making it a great wrap option.

Caprese Skewers

A fresh and simple snack with cherry tomatoes, mozzarella, and basil, drizzled with balsamic glaze.

Servings: 4 | Prep Time: 10 mins | Cook Time: 0 mins | Carbs per Serving : 5g

NUTRIENT CONTENT (PER SERVING):

- Calories: 100
- Total Fat: 7g
- Protein: 5g
- Carbohydrates: 5g
- Sugars: 3g
- Fiber: 1g
- Sodium: 150mg

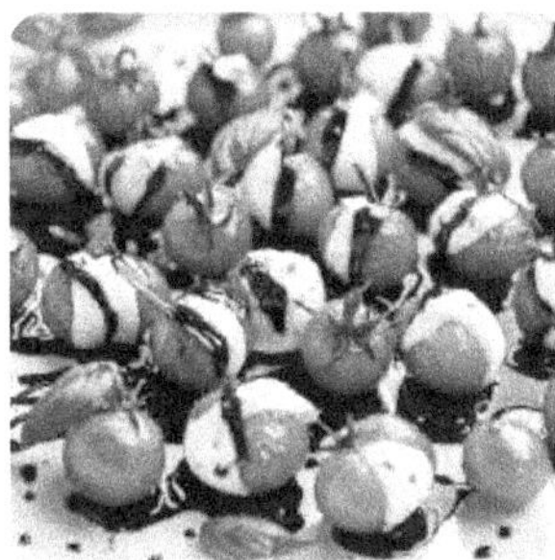

Ingredients

- Thread cherry tomatoes, mozzarella balls, and basil leaves onto skewers.
- Drizzle with balsamic glaze and season with salt and pepper.
- Serve immediately.

Directions

1. Preheat the oven to 350°F (175°C).
2. In a bowl, combine the mixed nuts, olive oil, chili powder, cumin, paprika, and salt.
3. Spread the nuts on a baking sheet in a single layer.
4. Bake for 10-12 minutes, stirring halfway through, until the nuts are toasted and fragrant.
5. Let cool before serving.

Ingredient Tips:

- Mozzarella: Provides protein and healthy fats, aiding in blood sugar control.
- Cherry Tomatoes: Low in calories and high in antioxidants.

Spinach & Feta Stuffed Mushrooms

Savory stuffed mushrooms with spinach and feta, perfect for a nutritious and flavorful appetizer.

Servings: 4 | Prep Time: 10mins | Cook Time: 20 mins | Carbs per Serving: 6g

NUTRIENT CONTENT (PER SERVING):

- Calories: 110
- Total Fat: 8g
- Protein: 5g
- Carbohydrates: 6g
- Sugars: 2g
- Fiber: 2g
- Sodium: 200mg

Ingredients

- 12 large mushroom caps
- 1 cup fresh spinach, chopped
- 1/2 cup crumbled feta cheese
- 2 cloves garlic, minced
- 2 tbsp olive oil
- Salt and pepper to taste

Directions

1. Preheat the oven to 375°F (190°C).
2. In a skillet, heat 1 tbsp of olive oil over medium heat. Add the garlic and spinach and cook until wilted.
3. In a bowl, combine the cooked spinach, feta cheese, and salt and pepper.
4. Stuff the mushroom caps with the spinach and feta mixture.
5. Place the stuffed mushrooms on a baking sheet and drizzle with the remaining olive oil.
6. Bake for 15-20 minutes, until the mushrooms are tender.
7. Serve immediately.

Ingredient Tips:

- Spinach: High in fiber and antioxidants, helping to manage blood sugar levels.
- Mushrooms: Low in calories and carbohydrates, making them a great base for stuffing.

Edamame with Sea Salt

A simple and protein-packed snack of steamed edamame sprinkled with sea salt.

Servings: 4 | Prep Time: 5 mins | Cook Time:5 mins | Carbs per Serving :9g

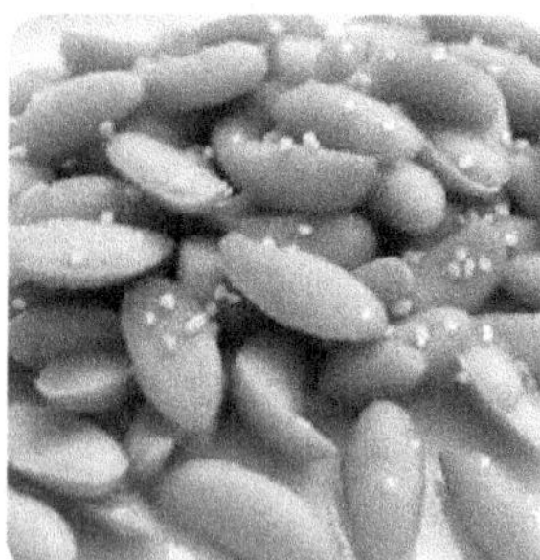

Ingredients

- 2 cups edamame in pods
- 1 tsp sea salt

Directions

1. Steam the edamame in pods for 5 minutes, until tender.
2. Drain and sprinkle with sea salt.
3. Serve immediately.

Ingredient Tips:

- Edamame: High in protein and fiber, aiding in blood sugar control.
- Sea Salt: Adds flavor without adding too many extra calories.

Guacamole with Bell Pepper Slices

Creamy homemade guacamole served with fresh bell pepper slices, perfect for a healthy and satisfying snack.

Servings: 4   Prep Time: 10mins | Cook Time: 0 mins | Carbs per Serving: 8g

Ingredients

- 2 ripe avocados
- 1 lime, juiced
- 1/4 cup red onion, diced
- 1 small tomato, diced
- 1 tbsp cilantro, chopped
- Salt and pepper to taste
- 1 bell pepper, sliced

Directions

1. In a bowl, mash the avocados with lime juice until smooth.
2. Stir in the red onion, tomato, cilantro, salt, and pepper.
3. Serve the guacamole with bell pepper slices.

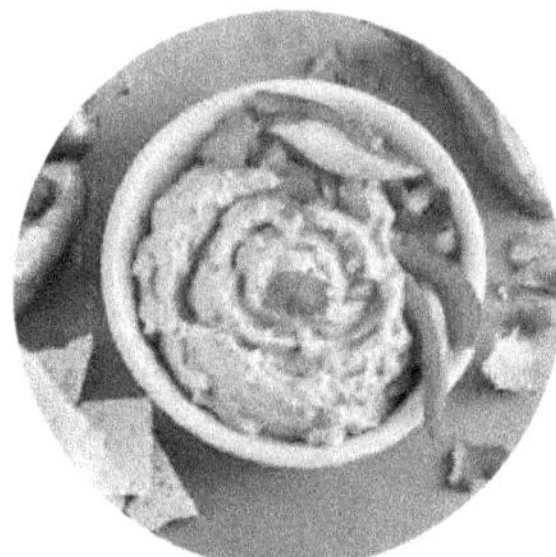

Ingredient Tips:

- Avocado: Provides healthy fats and fiber, aiding in blood sugar control.
- Bell Pepper: Low in calories and high in vitamins, making it a great dipping option.

Chapter Ten

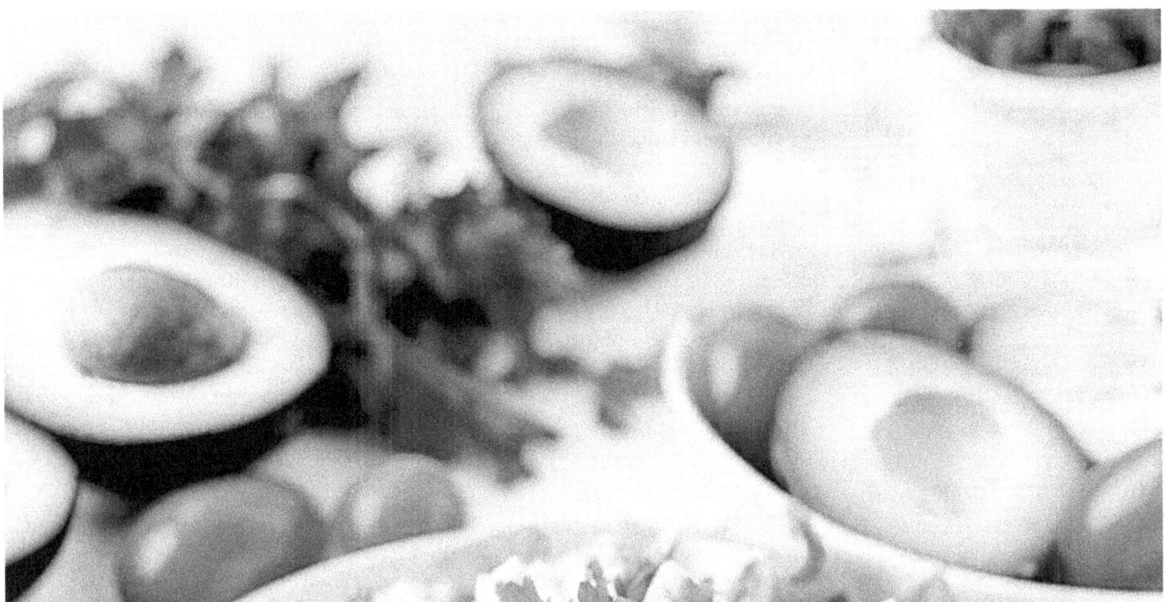

Salads and Sides Recipes

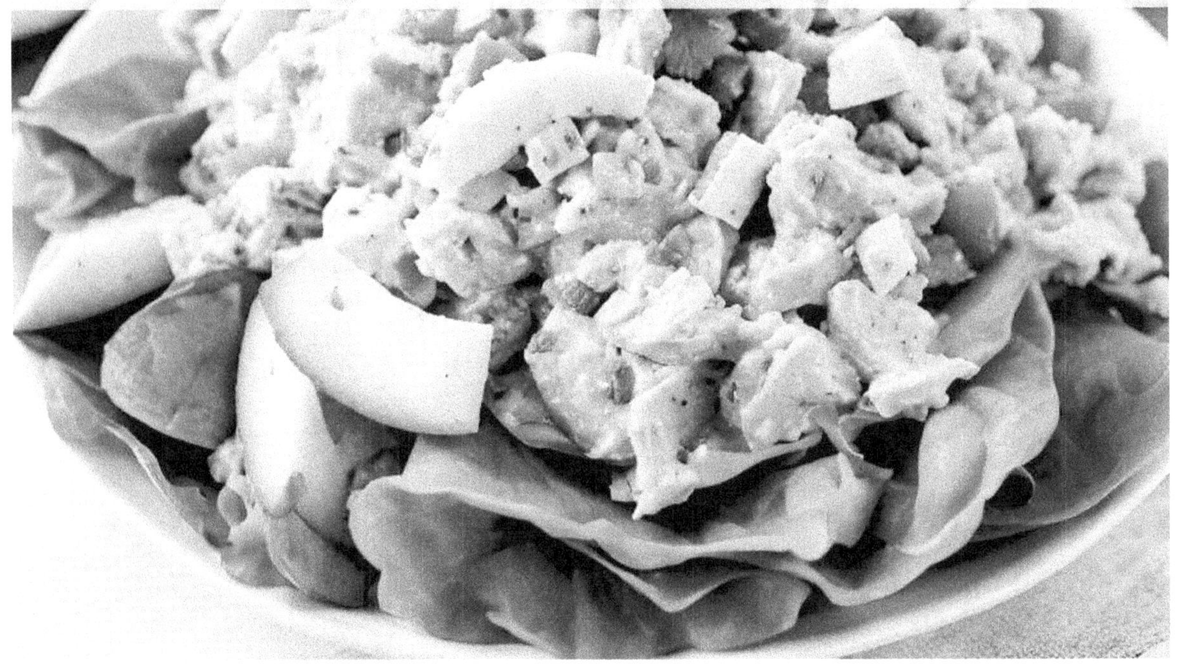

Grilled Chicken and Spinach Salad

A simple and delicious grilled chicken salad with fresh spinach and avocado, perfect for a light and satisfying meal.

Servings: 2 | Prep Time: 10 mins | Cook Time: 15 mins | Carbs per Serving :8g

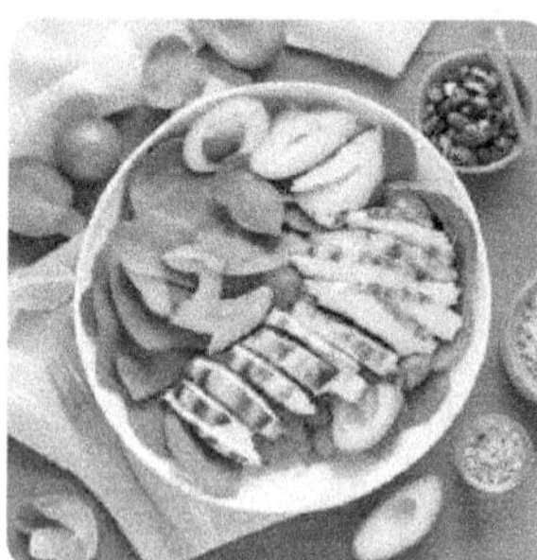

Ingredients

- 2 chicken breasts
- 4 cups fresh spinach leaves
- 1 avocado, sliced
- 1/2 cup cherry tomatoes, halved
- 1/4 cup red onion, thinly sliced
- 2 tbsp olive oil
- 1 tbsp balsamic vinegar
- Salt and pepper to taste

Directions

1. Season the chicken breasts with salt and pepper.
2. Grill the chicken over medium heat until cooked through, about 5-7 minutes per side. Let rest, then slice.
3. In a large bowl, combine the spinach, avocado, cherry tomatoes, and red onion.
4. Top with sliced grilled chicken.
5. In a small bowl, whisk together the olive oil and balsamic vinegar.
6. Drizzle the dressing over the salad and toss to combine.
7. Serve immediately.

Ingredient Tips:

- Chicken Breast: Lean protein that helps manage blood sugar levels.
- Spinach: High in fiber and low in carbs, excellent for blood sugar control.

Lentil and Tomato Salad

A hearty and protein-rich salad with lentils, fresh tomatoes, and a zesty lemon dressing.

Servings: 4   Prep Time: 10mins | Cook Time: 20 mins | Carbs per Serving: 20g

Ingredients

- 1 cup cooked lentils
- 2 cups cherry tomatoes, halved
- 1/2 cup cucumber, diced
- 1/4 cup red onion, finely chopped
- 2 tbsp olive oil
- 1 tbsp lemon juice
- Salt and pepper to taste
- Fresh parsley for garnish

Directions

1. In a large bowl, combine the cooked lentils, cherry tomatoes, cucumber, and red onion.
2. In a small bowl, whisk together the olive oil, lemon juice, salt, and pepper.
3. Pour the dressing over the lentil mixture and toss to combine.
4. Garnish with fresh parsley and serve.

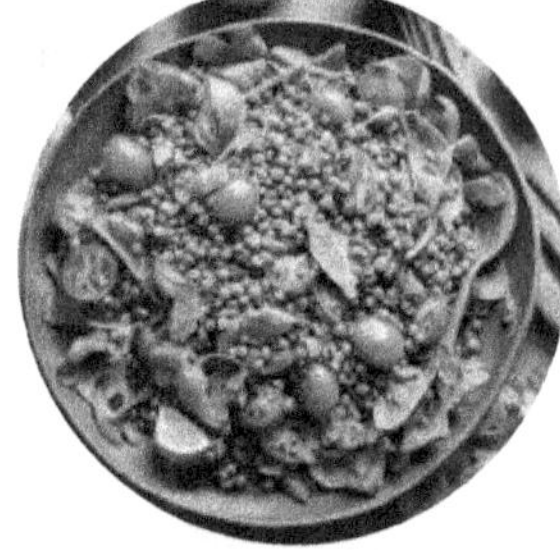

Ingredient Tips:

- Lentils: High in protein and fiber, making them great for managing blood sugar levels.
- Tomatoes: Low glycemic index and rich in vitamins.

Quinoa and Kale Salad

A nutrient-dense quinoa and kale salad with avocado and a tangy lemon vinaigrette.

Servings: 4 | Prep Time: 10 mins | Cook Time: 20 mins | Carbs per Serving 22g

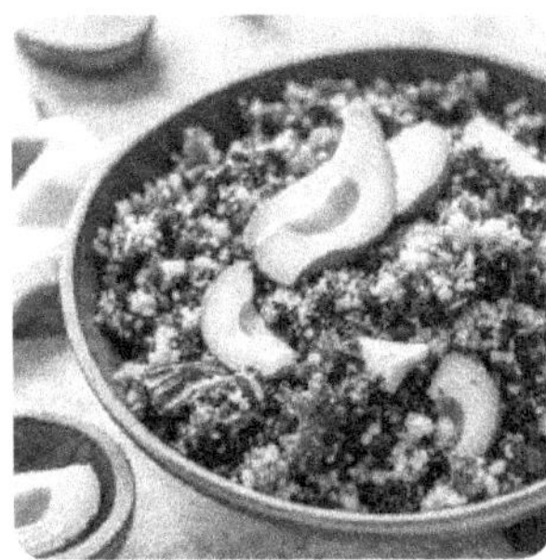

Ingredients

- 1 cup cooked quinoa
- 2 cups chopped kale
- 1 avocado, diced
- 1/2 cup cherry tomatoes, halved
- 1/4 cup red onion, thinly sliced
- 2 tbsp olive oil
- 1 tbsp lemon juice
- Salt and pepper to taste

Directions

1. In a large bowl, combine the cooked quinoa, kale, avocado, cherry tomatoes, and red onion.
2. In a small bowl, whisk together the olive oil, lemon juice, salt, and pepper.
3. Pour the dressing over the quinoa mixture and toss to combine.
4. Serve immediately.

Ingredient Tips:

- Quinoa: High in protein and fiber, helping to stabilize blood sugar levels.
- Kale: Low in carbs and high in vitamins and fiber.

Tuna and Avocado Salad

A simple and delicious tuna salad with creamy avocado and fresh vegetables, perfect for a quick and healthy meal.

Servings: 2   Prep Time: 10mins | Cook Time: 0 mins | Carbs per serving: 8g

Ingredients

- 1 can tuna in water, drained
- 1 avocado, diced
- 1/2 cup cherry tomatoes, halved
- 1/4 cup red onion, diced
- 2 tbsp olive oil
- 1 tbsp lemon juice
- Salt and pepper to taste

Directions

1. In a large bowl, combine the tuna, avocado, cherry tomatoes, and red onion.
2. In a small bowl, whisk together the olive oil, lemon juice, salt, and pepper.
3. Pour the dressing over the tuna mixture and toss to combine.
4. Serve immediately.

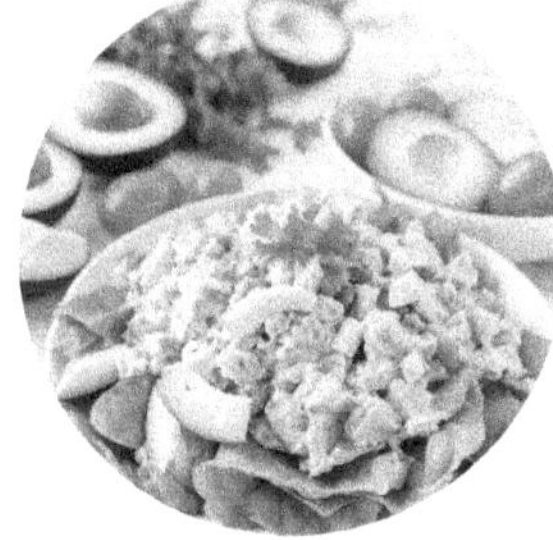

Ingredient Tips:

- Tuna: High in protein and omega-3 fatty acids, aiding in blood sugar management and heart health.
- Avocado: Provides healthy fats and fiber, aiding in blood sugar control.

Greek Yogurt and Cucumber Salad

A refreshing and protein-packed salad with Greek yogurt, cucumbers, and fresh dill.

Servings: 2 | Prep Time: 10 mins | Cook Time: 0 mins | Carbs per Serving 10g

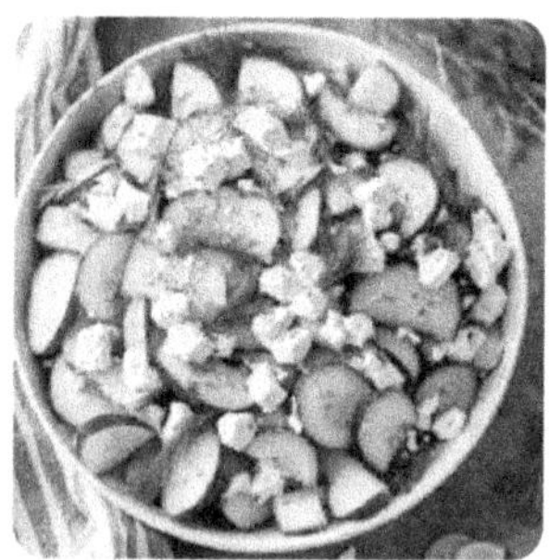

Ingredients

- 1 cup Greek yogurt
- 1 large cucumber, sliced
- 1/4 cup red onion, thinly sliced
- 1 tbsp fresh dill, chopped
- 1 tbsp lemon juice
- Salt and pepper to taste

Directions

1. In a large bowl, combine the Greek yogurt, cucumber, red onion, and fresh dill.
2. Add the lemon juice, salt, and pepper, and mix well.
3. Serve immediately or chill in the refrigerator before serving.

Ingredient Tips:

- Greek Yogurt: High in protein and probiotics, beneficial for gut health and blood sugar control.
- Cucumber: Low in calories and carbs, hydrating and refreshing.

Chickpea and Spinach Salad

A hearty and nutritious salad with chickpeas, fresh spinach, and a lemon-tahini dressing.

Servings: 4   Prep Time: 10mins | Cook Time: 0 mins | Carbs per serving: 18g

Ingredients

- 1 can chickpeas, drained and rinsed
- 4 cups fresh spinach leaves
- 1/2 cup cherry tomatoes, halved
- 1/4 cup red onion, thinly sliced
- 2 tbsp tahini
- 1 tbsp lemon juice
- 1 tbsp olive oil
- Salt and pepper to taste
-

Directions

1. In a large bowl, combine the chickpeas, spinach, cherry tomatoes, and red onion.
2. In a small bowl, whisk together the tahini, lemon juice, olive oil, salt, and pepper.
3. Pour the dressing over the salad and toss to combine.
4. Serve immediately

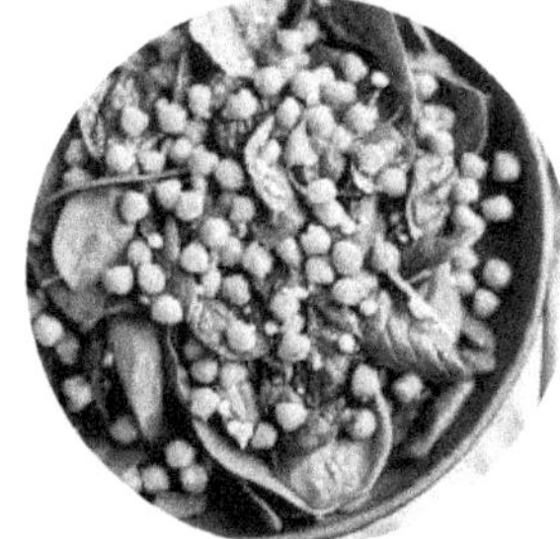

Ingredient Tips:

- Chickpeas: High in protein and fiber, making them excellent for blood sugar control.
- Spinach: Packed with vitamins and fiber, low in carbs.

Shrimp and Avocado Salad

A light and flavorful salad with shrimp, avocado, and a lime-cilantro dressing.

Servings: 4 | Prep Time: 10 mins | Cook Time: 0 mins | Carbs per Serving: 6g

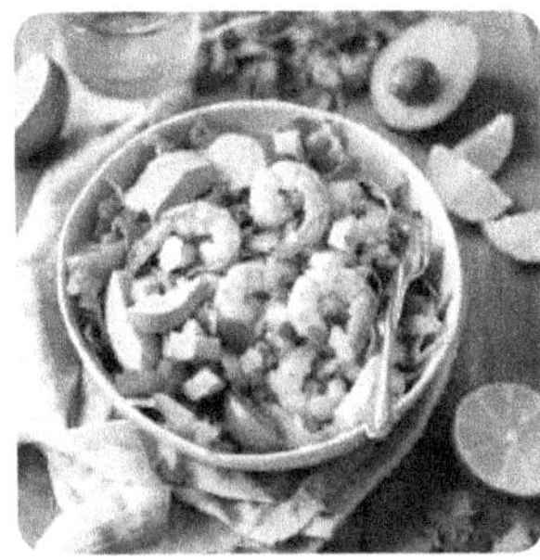

Ingredients

- 1 lb shrimp, cooked and peeled
- 1 avocado, diced
- 1/2 cup cherry tomatoes, halved
- 1/4 cup red onion, diced
- 2 tbsp olive oil
- 1 tbsp lime juice
- Fresh cilantro for garnish
- Salt and pepper to taste

Directions

1. In a large bowl, combine the shrimp, avocado, cherry tomatoes, and red onion.
2. In a small bowl, whisk together the olive oil, lime juice, salt, and pepper.
3. Pour the dressing over the shrimp mixture and toss to combine.
4. Garnish with fresh cilantro and serve immediately.

Ingredient Tips:

- Shrimp: High in protein and low in carbs, great for maintaining blood sugar levels.
- Avocado: Provides healthy fats and fiber, aiding in blood sugar control.

Turkey and Berry Salad

A savory and slightly sweet salad with turkey breast and fresh berries, perfect for a balanced and tasty meal.

Servings: 2 | Prep Time: 10mins | Cook Time: 0 mins | Carbs per serving: 10g

Ingredients

- 2 cups mixed greens
- 1 cup cooked turkey breast, sliced
- 1/2 cup fresh berries (blueberries, strawberries, or raspberries)
- 1/4 cup red onion, thinly sliced
- 2 tbsp olive oil
- 1 tbsp balsamic vinegar
- Salt and pepper to taste

Directions

1. In a large bowl, combine the mixed greens, turkey breast, fresh berries, and red onion.
2. In a small bowl, whisk together the olive oil, balsamic vinegar, salt, and pepper.
3. Pour the dressing over the salad and toss to combine.
4. Serve immediately.

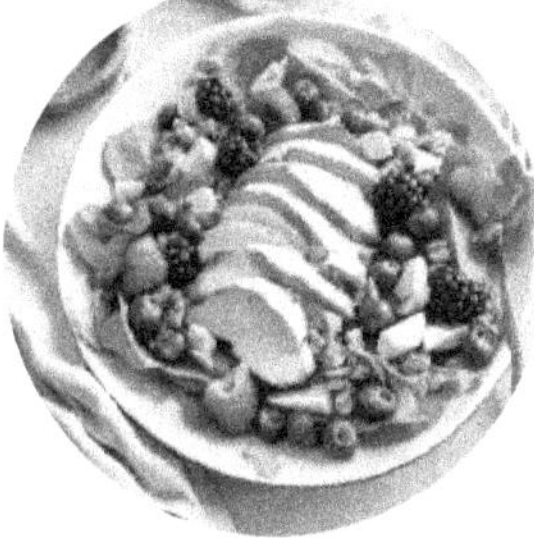

Ingredient Tips:

- Turkey Breast: Lean protein that helps keep blood sugar levels stable.
- Berries: Low glycemic index fruits that add natural sweetness and fiber.

Bean and Corn Salad

A colorful and fiber-rich salad with black beans, corn, and a tangy lime dressing.

Servings: 4 | Prep Time: 10 mins | Cook Time: 0 mins | Carbs per Serving: 22g

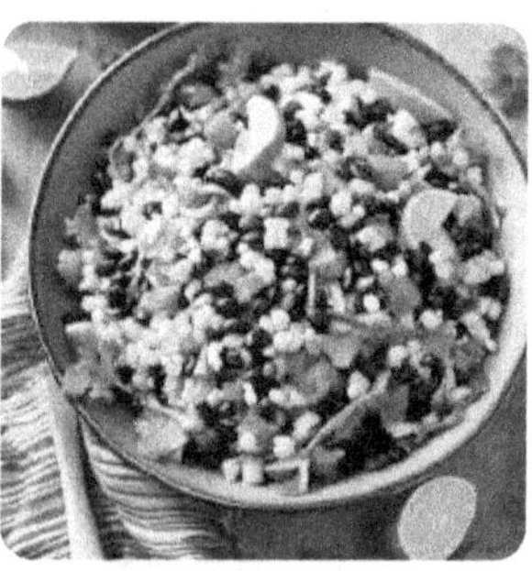

Ingredients

- 1 can black beans, drained and rinsed
- 1 cup corn kernels (fresh or frozen)
- 1/2 cup cherry tomatoes, halved
- 1/4 cup red onion, diced
- 2 tbsp olive oil
- 1 tbsp lime juice
- Fresh cilantro for garnish
- Salt and pepper to taste

Directions

1. In a large bowl, combine the black beans, corn, cherry tomatoes, and red onion.
2. In a small bowl, whisk together the olive oil, lime juice, salt, and pepper.
3. Pour the dressing over the bean mixture and toss to combine.
4. Garnish with fresh cilantro and serve.

Ingredient Tips:

- Black Beans: High in protein and fiber, helping to manage blood sugar levels.
- Corn: Provides fiber and essential vitamins, though should be consumed in moderation due to its carbohydrate content.

Egg and Asparagus Salad

A fresh and satisfying salad with hard-boiled eggs and tender asparagus, topped with a mustard vinaigrette.

Servings: 2   Prep Time: 10mins | Cook Time: 10 mins | Carbs per serving: 8g

Ingredients

- 4 hard-boiled eggs, sliced
- 1 bunch asparagus, trimmed and blanched
- 2 cups mixed greens
- 1/4 cup red onion, thinly sliced
- 2 tbsp olive oil
- 1 tbsp Dijon mustard
- 1 tbsp lemon juice
- Salt and pepper to taste

Directions

1. In a large bowl, combine the mixed greens, blanched asparagus, and red onion.
2. Top with sliced hard-boiled eggs.
3. In a small bowl, whisk together the olive oil, Dijon mustard, lemon juice, salt, and pepper.
4. Pour the dressing over the salad and toss to combine.
5. Serve immediately.

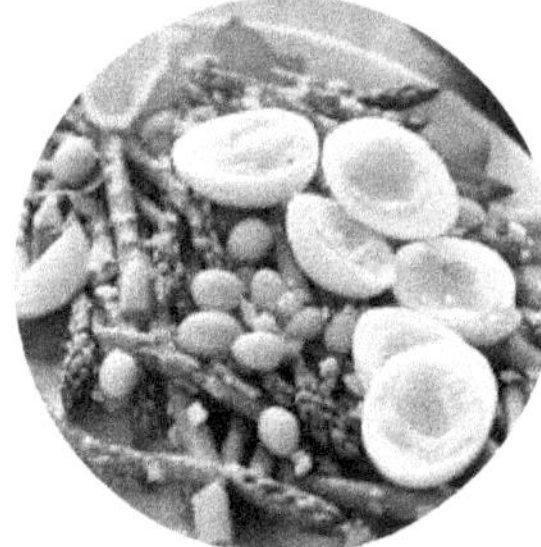

Ingredient Tips:

- Eggs: High in protein and healthy fats, great for blood sugar management.
- Asparagus: Low in calories and carbs, high in vitamins and fiber.

Chapter Eleven

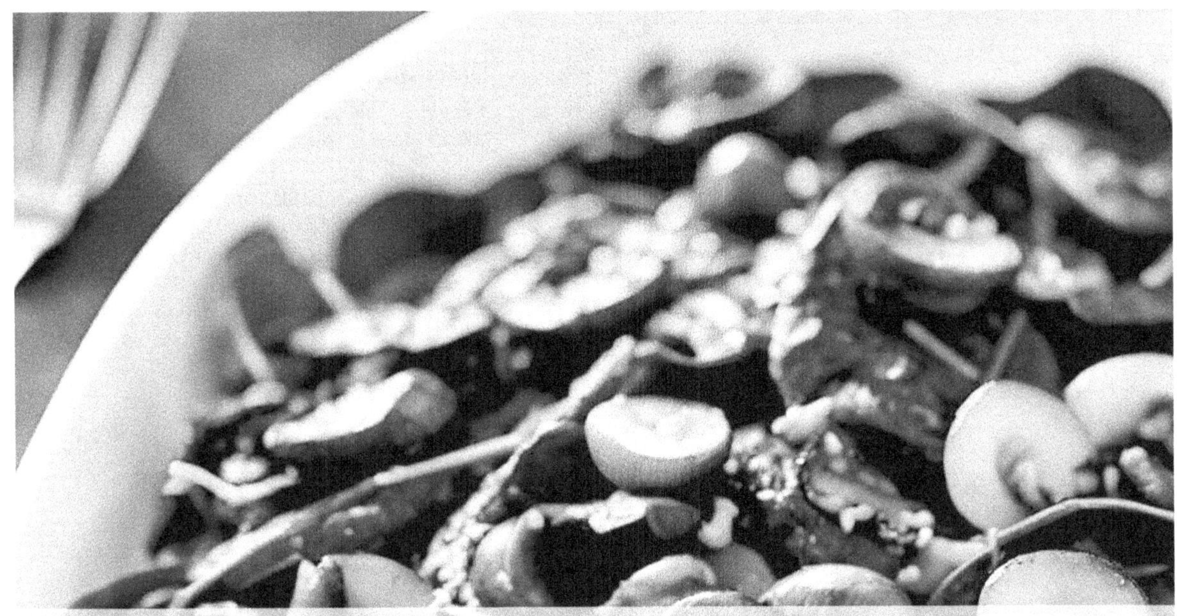

Vegetarian Options Recipes

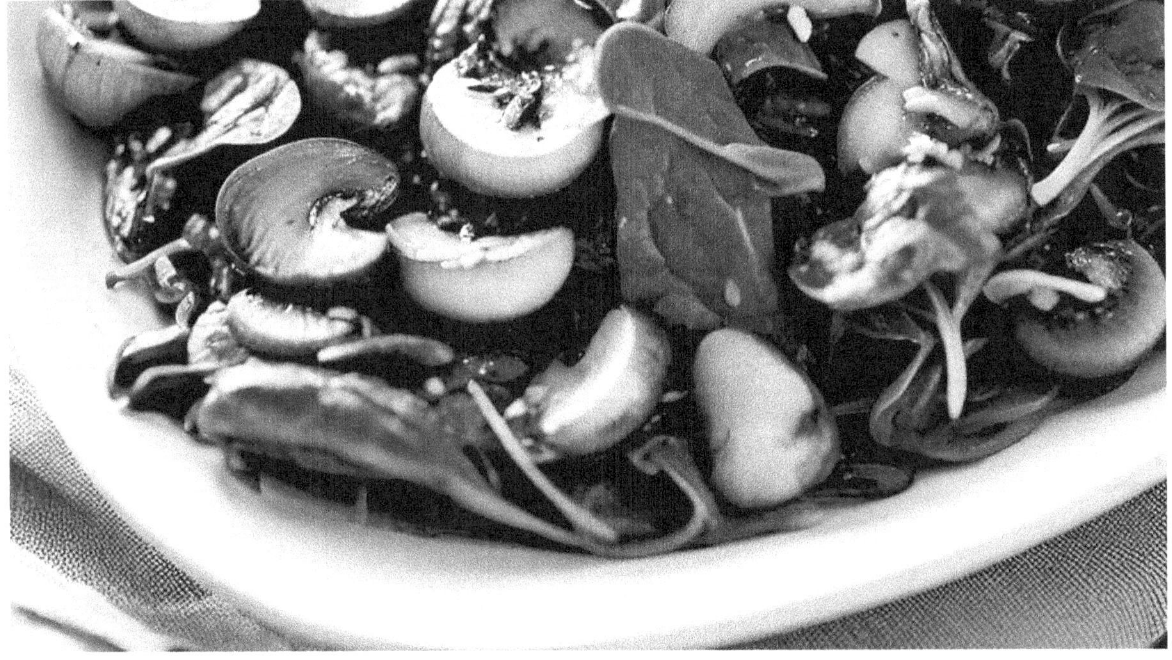

Roasted Brussels Sprouts with Almonds

Crispy roasted Brussels sprouts with a crunchy almond topping, perfect for a nutritious side dish.

Servings: 4 | Prep Time: 5 mins | Cook Time: 25 mins | Carbs per Serving: 8g

NUTRIENT CONTENT (PER SERVING):

- Calories: 140
- Total Fat: 10g
- Protein: 4g
- Carbohydrates: 8g
- Sugars: 2g
- Fiber: 4g
- Sodium: 150mg

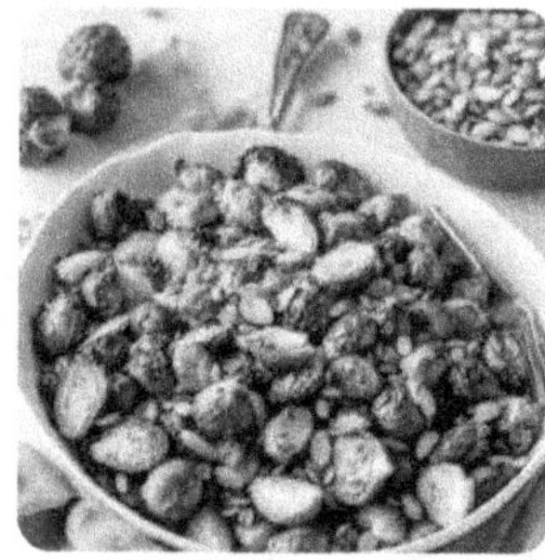

Ingredients

- 1 lb Brussels sprouts, halved
- 2 tbsp olive oil
- 1/4 cup sliced almonds
- Salt and pepper to taste

Directions

1. Preheat the oven to 400°F (200°C).
2. Toss the Brussels sprouts with olive oil, salt, and pepper.
3. Spread the Brussels sprouts on a baking sheet in a single layer.
4. Roast for 20-25 minutes, or until crispy and golden brown.
5. In the last 5 minutes of roasting, sprinkle the almonds over the Brussels sprouts.
6. Serve hot.

Ingredient Tips:

- Brussels Sprouts: Low in calories and high in fiber, making them great for blood sugar control.
- Almonds: Provide healthy fats and protein, aiding in satiety and blood sugar management.

Spinach and Mushroom Sauté

A quick and easy sauté of spinach and mushrooms with garlic, perfect for a healthy side dish.

Servings: 2   Prep Time: 5 mins | Cook Time: 10 mins | Carbs per serving: 5g

NUTRIENT CONTENT (PER SERVING):

- Calories: 110
- Total Fat: 10g
- Protein: 2g
- Carbohydrates: 5g
- Sugars: 2g
- Fiber: 2g
- Sodium: 200mg

Ingredients

- 2 cups fresh spinach
- 1 cup sliced mushrooms
- 2 cloves garlic, minced
- 2 tbsp olive oil
- Salt and pepper to taste

Directions

1. In a large skillet, heat the olive oil over medium heat.
2. Add the garlic and sauté until fragrant.
3. Add the mushrooms and cook until tender.
4. Add the spinach and cook until wilted.
5. Season with salt and pepper to taste and serve hot.

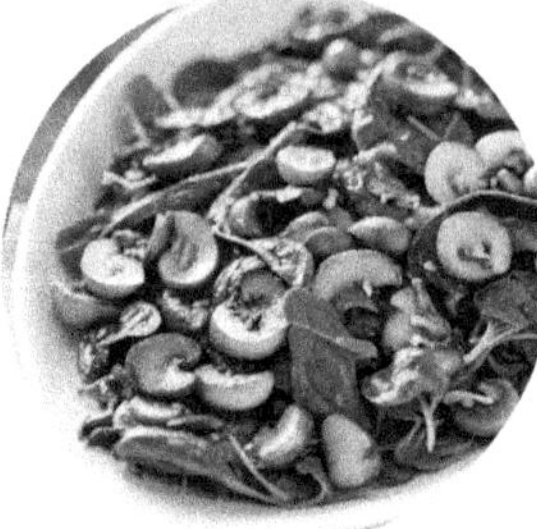

Ingredient Tips:

- Spinach: High in fiber and low in calories, making it excellent for blood sugar control.
- Mushrooms: Low in calories and provide a good amount of fiber and nutrients.

Cauliflower Rice with Herbs

A low-carb alternative to traditional rice, flavored with fresh herbs for a light and tasty side dish.

Servings: 4 | Prep Time: 10 mins | Cook Time: 7 mins | Carbs per Serving: 6g

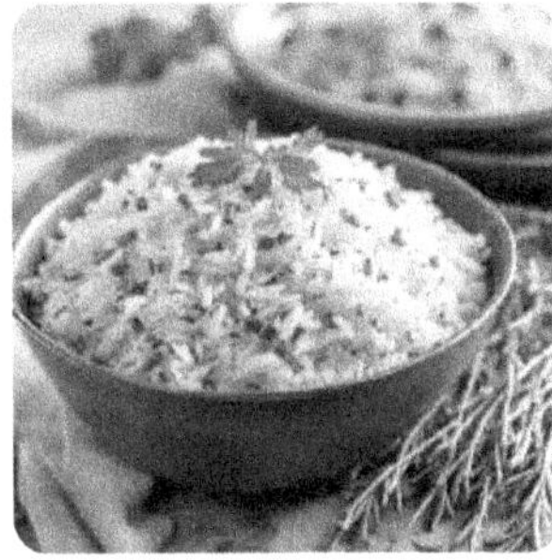

Ingredients

- 1 medium cauliflower, grated to resemble rice
- 2 tbsp olive oil
- 1/4 cup chopped fresh parsley
- 1/4 cup chopped fresh cilantro
- Salt and pepper to taste

Directions

1. In a large skillet, heat the olive oil over medium heat.
2. Add the grated cauliflower and cook for 5-7 minutes, or until tender.
3. Stir in the chopped parsley and cilantro.
4. Season with salt and pepper to taste and serve hot.

Ingredient Tips:

- Cauliflower: A low-carb vegetable that helps keep carbohydrate intake low.
- Herbs: Add flavor without adding calories or sugar.

Baked Zucchini Fries

Crispy and delicious zucchini fries baked to perfection, a great low-carb alternative to traditional fries.

Servings: 4   Prep Time: 10 mins | Cook Time: 25 mins | Carbs per serving: 7g

Ingredients

- 2 medium zucchinis, cut into fries
- 1/4 cup grated Parmesan cheese
- 1/4 cup almond flour
- 2 tbsp olive oil
- 1 tsp garlic powder
- Salt and pepper to taste

Directions

1. Preheat the oven to 425°F (220°C).
2. In a bowl, toss the zucchini fries with olive oil.
3. In another bowl, combine the Parmesan cheese, almond flour, garlic powder, salt, and pepper.
4. Coat the zucchini fries in the cheese mixture.
5. Place the zucchini fries on a baking sheet lined with parchment paper.
6. Bake for 20-25 minutes, or until golden and crispy.
7. Serve hot.

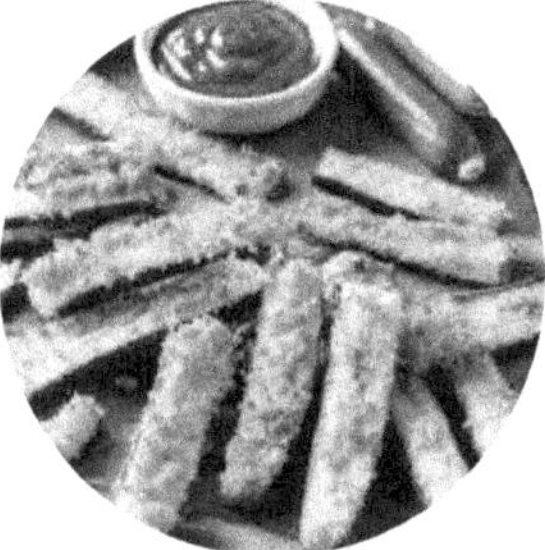

Ingredient Tips:

- Zucchini: Low in carbs and high in fiber, making it excellent for blood sugar control.
- Almond Flour: A low-carb alternative to traditional flour, adding healthy fats and protein.

Roasted Asparagus with Lemon and Parmesan

Simple and flavorful roasted asparagus with a touch of lemon and Parmesan cheese, perfect for a light side dish.

Servings: 4 | Prep Time: 5 mins | Cook Time: 20 mins | Carbs per Serving: 4g

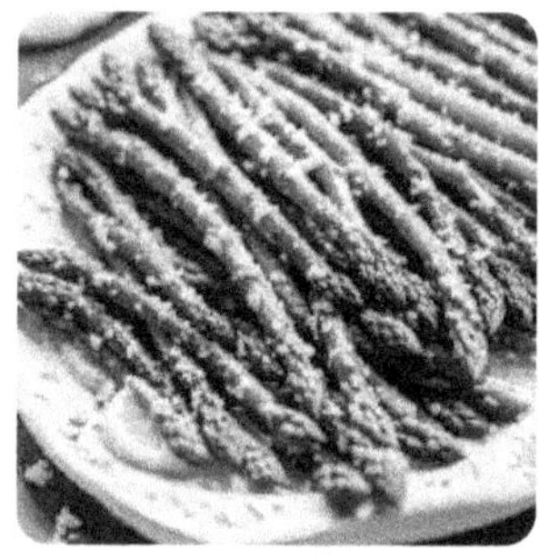

Ingredients

- 1 lb asparagus, trimmed
- 2 tbsp olive oil
- 1/4 cup grated Parmesan cheese
- 1 tbsp lemon juice
- Salt and pepper to taste

Directions

1. Preheat the oven to 400°F (200°C).
2. Toss the asparagus with olive oil, salt, and pepper.
3. Spread the asparagus on a baking sheet in a single layer.
4. Roast for 15-20 minutes, or until tender and slightly crispy.
5. Drizzle with lemon juice and sprinkle with Parmesan cheese.
6. Serve hot.

Ingredient Tips:

- Asparagus: Low in calories and high in fiber, making it great for blood sugar control.
- Parmesan Cheese: Adds flavor and protein without adding many carbs.

Garlic Green Beans

A simple and tasty side dish of green beans sautéed with garlic, perfect for any meal.

Servings: 4   Prep Time: 5 mins | Cook Time: 7 mins | Carbs per serving: 6g

Ingredients

- 1 lb green beans, trimmed
- 2 cloves garlic, minced
- 2 tbsp olive oil
- Salt and pepper to taste

Directions

1. In a large skillet, heat the olive oil over medium heat.
2. Add the garlic and sauté until fragrant.
3. Add the green beans and cook until tender-crisp, about 5-7 minutes.
4. Season with salt and pepper to taste and serve hot.

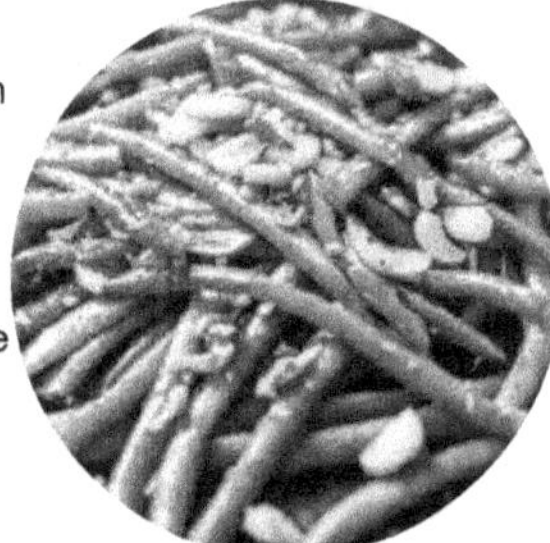

Ingredient Tips:

- Green Beans: High in fiber and low in calories, making them excellent for blood sugar control.
- Garlic: Adds flavor without adding calories or carbs.

Cucumber and Tomato Salad

A refreshing and simple salad of cucumbers and tomatoes with a light vinaigrette, perfect for a quick side dish.

Servings: 4 | Prep Time: 10 mins | Cook Time: 0 mins | Carbs per Serving: 5g

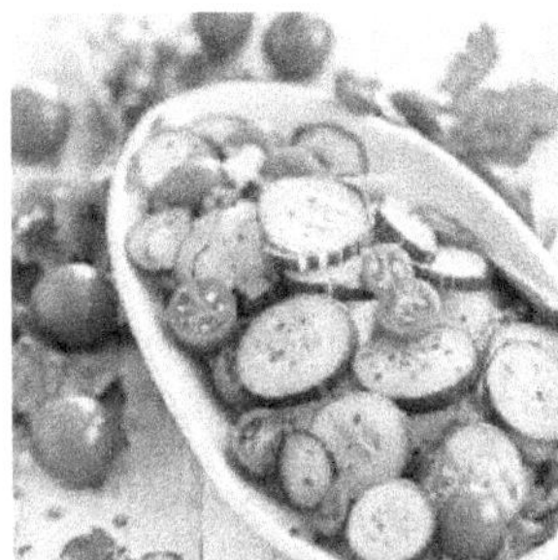

Ingredients

- 2 cups cucumber, sliced
- 1 cup cherry tomatoes, halved
- 1/4 cup red onion, thinly sliced
- 2 tbsp olive oil
- 1 tbsp red wine vinegar
- Salt and pepper to taste

Directions

1. In a large bowl, combine the cucumber, cherry tomatoes, and red onion.
2. In a small bowl, whisk together the olive oil, red wine vinegar, salt, and pepper.
3. Pour the dressing over the salad and toss to combine.
4. Serve immediately.

Ingredient Tips:

- Cucumber: Low in calories and high in water content, making it great for hydration and blood sugar control.
- Tomatoes: Provide vitamins and fiber, aiding in blood sugar management.

Baked Eggplant with Tahini

A savory baked eggplant dish topped with creamy tahini sauce, perfect for a flavorful side.

Servings: 4 | Prep Time: 10 mins | Cook Time: 25 mins | Carbs per serving: 10g

Ingredients

- 1 large eggplant, sliced
- 2 tbsp olive oil
- 1/4 cup tahini
- 1 tbsp lemon juice
- 1 clove garlic, minced
- Salt and pepper to taste
- Fresh parsley for garnish

Directions

1. Preheat the oven to 400°F (200°C).
2. Brush the eggplant slices with olive oil and season with salt and pepper.
3. Place on a baking sheet and bake for 20-25 minutes, or until tender.
4. In a small bowl, whisk together the tahini, lemon juice, garlic, salt, and pepper.
5. Drizzle the tahini sauce over the baked eggplant.
6. Garnish with fresh parsley and serve hot.

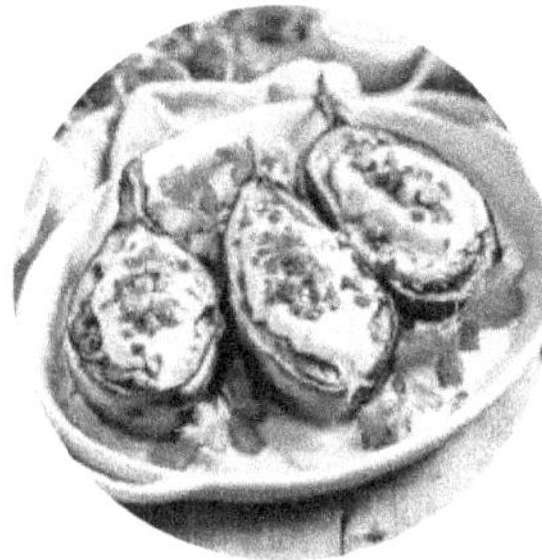

Ingredient Tips:

- Eggplant: Low in calories and high in fiber, making it great for blood sugar control.
- Tahini: Provides healthy fats and protein, aiding in satiety and blood sugar management.

Roasted Carrot and Lentil Salad

A hearty salad of roasted carrots and lentils with a tangy dressing, perfect for a nutritious side dish.

Servings: 4 | Prep Time: 10 mins | Cook Time: 25 mins | Carbs per Serving: 20g

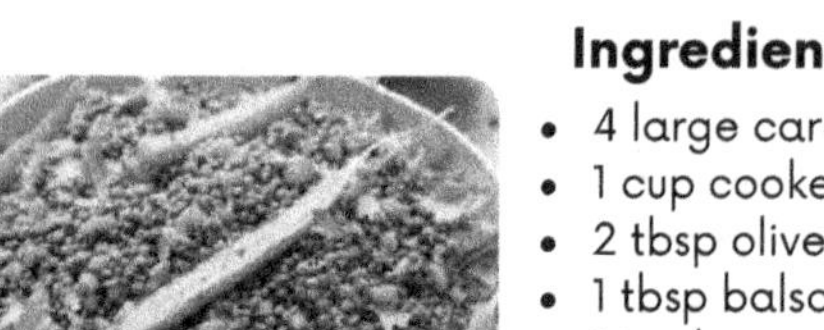

Ingredients

- 4 large carrots, sliced
- 1 cup cooked lentils
- 2 tbsp olive oil
- 1 tbsp balsamic vinegar
- 1 tsp honey (optional)
- Salt and pepper to taste
- Fresh parsley for garnish

Directions

1. Preheat the oven to 400°F (200°C).
2. Toss the carrot slices with 1 tbsp of olive oil, salt, and pepper.
3. Spread the carrots on a baking sheet and roast for 20-25 minutes, or until tender.
4. In a large bowl, combine the roasted carrots and cooked lentils.
5. In a small bowl, whisk together the remaining olive oil, balsamic vinegar, and honey (if using).
6. Pour the dressing over the salad and toss to combine.
7. Garnish with fresh parsley and serve hot or at room temperature.

Ingredient Tips:

- Carrots: Provide vitamins and fiber, aiding in blood sugar management.
- Lentils: High in protein and fiber, helping to manage blood sugar levels.

Stuffed Bell Peppers with Quinoa

Colorful bell peppers stuffed with a flavorful quinoa and vegetable filling, perfect for a healthy and satisfying side.

Servings: 4   Prep Time: 15 mins | Cook Time: 30 mins | Carbs per serving: 25g

Ingredients

- 4 large bell peppers, tops cut off and seeds removed
- 1 cup cooked quinoa
- 1 cup diced tomatoes
- 1/2 cup black beans, drained and rinsed
- 1/2 cup corn kernels
- 1/4 cup chopped cilantro
- 2 tbsp olive oil
- 1 tsp cumin
- Salt and pepper to taste

Directions

1. Preheat the oven to 375°F (190°C).
2. In a large bowl, combine the cooked quinoa, diced tomatoes, black beans, corn, cilantro, olive oil, cumin, salt, and pepper.
3. Stuff the bell peppers with the quinoa mixture.
4. Place the stuffed peppers in a baking dish and cover with foil.
5. Bake for 25-30 minutes, or until the peppers are tender.
6. Serve hot.

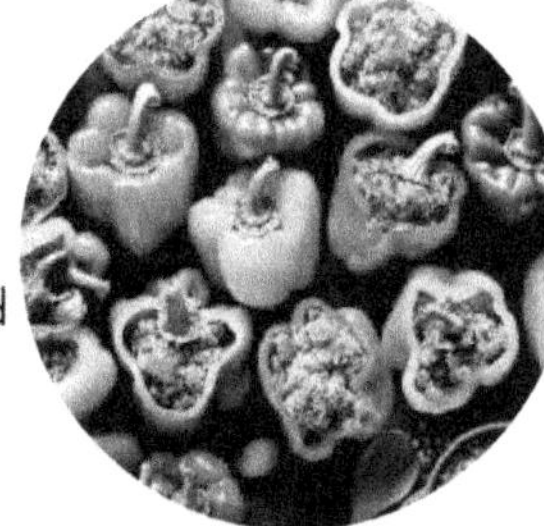

Ingredient Tips:

- Bell Peppers: Low in calories and high in fiber and vitamins, making them great for blood sugar control.
- Quinoa: A whole grain that is high in protein and fiber, aiding in satiety and blood sugar management.

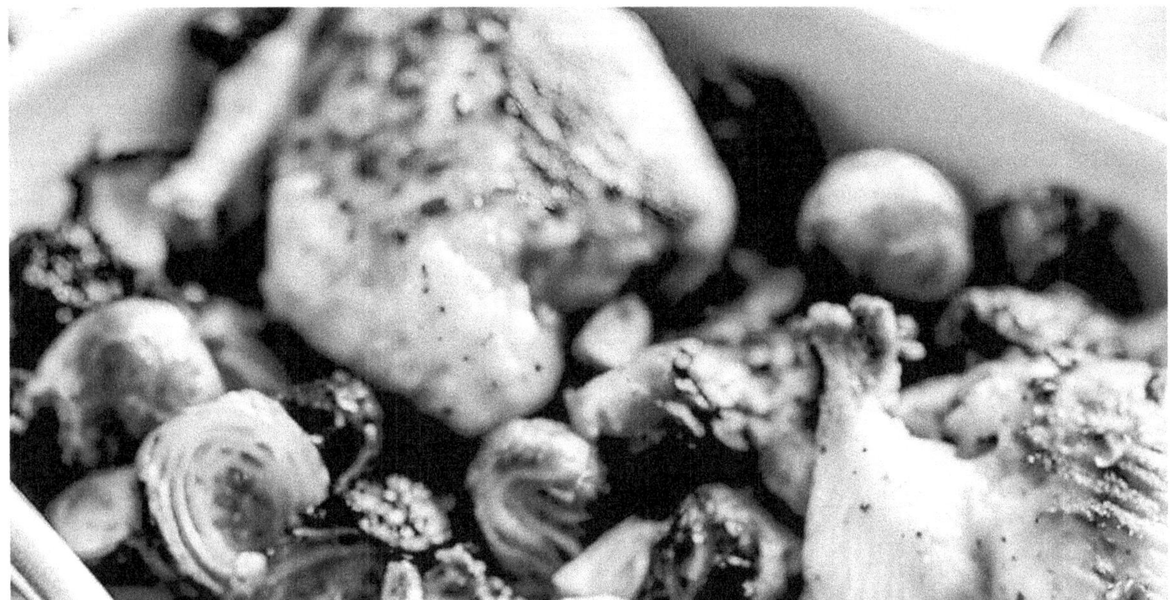

Chapter Twelve

Chicken & Turkey Options Recipes

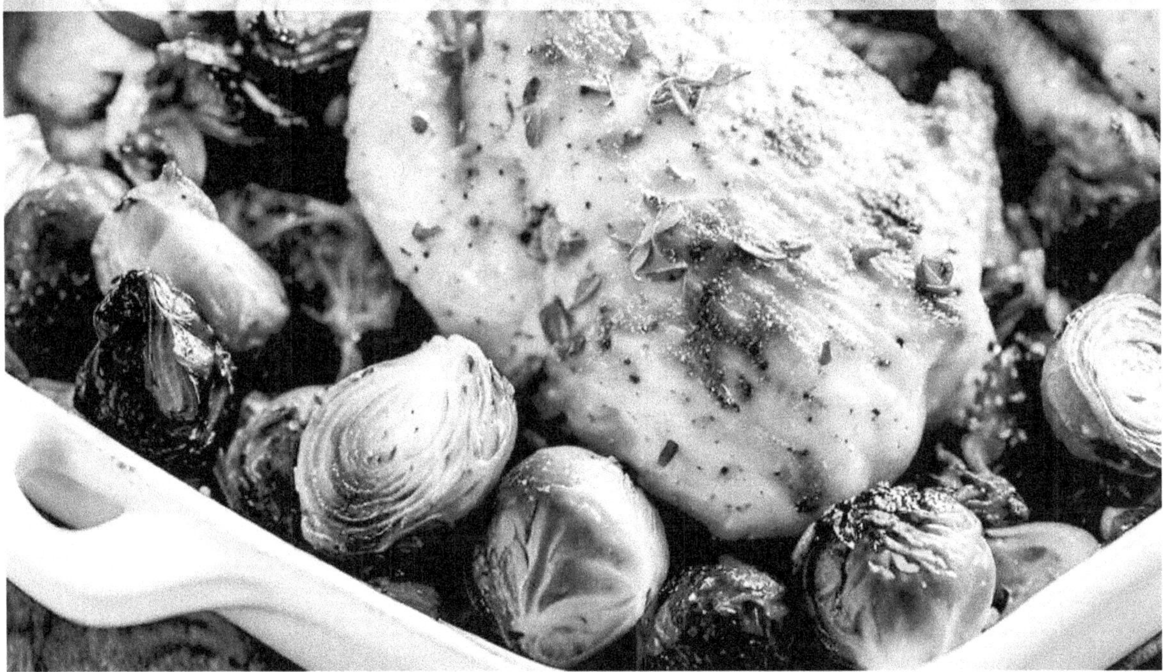

Lemon Herb Chicken Breast

A light and flavorful chicken breast marinated in lemon juice and herbs, perfect for a quick and healthy lunch or dinner.

Servings: 2 | Prep Time: 10 mins | Cook Time: 15 mins | Carbs per Serving: 2g

- Calories: 280
- Total Fat: 14g
- Protein: 34g
- Carbohydrates: 2g
- Sugars: 0g
- Fiber: 1g
- Sodium: 150mg

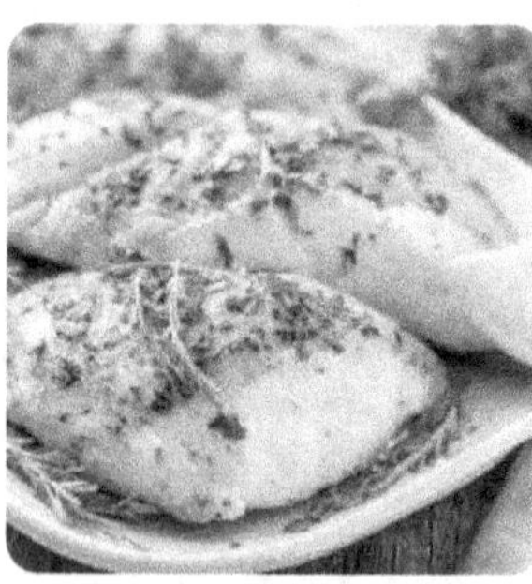

Ingredients

- 2 chicken breasts
- 2 tbsp olive oil
- Juice of 1 lemon
- 2 cloves garlic, minced
- 1 tsp dried oregano
- 1 tsp dried thyme
- Salt and pepper to taste

Directions

1. In a bowl, combine the olive oil, lemon juice, garlic, oregano, thyme, salt, and pepper.
2. Add the chicken breasts and marinate for at least 30 minutes.
3. Preheat the grill to medium-high heat.
4. Grill the chicken breasts for 5-7 minutes per side, or until cooked through.
5. Let rest for a few minutes before slicing and serving.

Ingredient Tips:

- Chicken Breast: A lean protein source that helps keep you full and stabilize blood sugar levels.
- Lemon Juice: Adds flavor without added sugar or calories.

Avocado Chicken Salad

A creamy and satisfying chicken salad with avocado and fresh vegetables, perfect for a nutritious lunch.

Servings: 2   Prep Time: 10 mins | Cook Time: 0 mins | Carbs per serving: 8g

NUTRIENT CONTENT (PER SERVING):

- Calories: 350
- Total Fat: 24g
- Protein: 28g
- Carbohydrates: 8g
- Sugars: 2g
- Fiber: 5g
- Sodium: 250mg

Ingredients

- 2 chicken breasts, cooked and shredded
- 1 avocado, diced
- 1/2 cup cherry tomatoes, halved
- 1/4 cup red onion, diced
- 2 tbsp olive oil
- 1 tbsp lime juice
- Salt and pepper to taste

Directions

1. In a large bowl, combine the shredded chicken, avocado, cherry tomatoes, and red onion.
2. In a small bowl, whisk together the olive oil, lime juice, salt, and pepper.
3. Pour the dressing over the chicken mixture and toss to combine.
4. Serve immediately or chill until ready to serve.

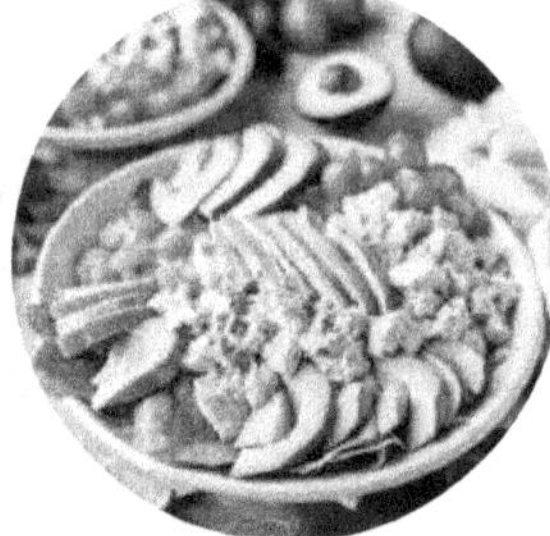

Ingredient Tips:

- Avocado: Provides healthy fats and fiber, aiding in blood sugar control.
- Chicken Breast: Lean and high in protein, helping to keep you full and manage blood sugar levels.

Spinach and Chicken Stuffed Peppers

Colorful bell peppers stuffed with a delicious mixture of chicken, spinach, and cheese, baked to perfection.

Servings: 4 | Prep Time: 15 mins | Cook Time: 25 mins | Carbs per Serving: 10g

NUTRIENT CONTENT (PER SERVING):

- Calories: 220
- Total Fat: 12g
- Protein: 20g
- Carbohydrates: 10g
- Sugars: 6g
- Fiber: 3g
- Sodium: 300mg

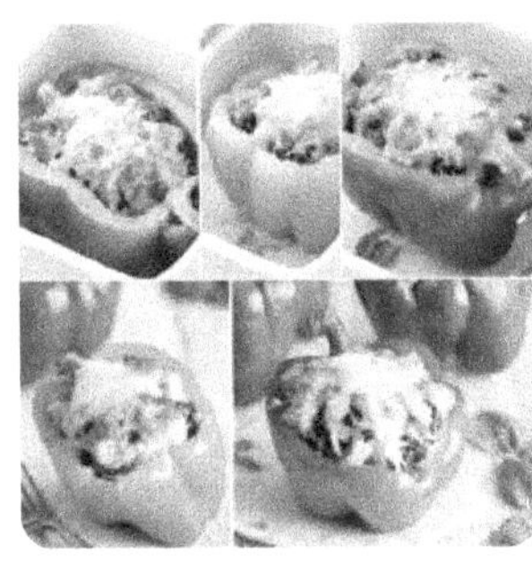

Ingredients

- 4 bell peppers, halved and seeded
- 2 chicken breasts, cooked and shredded
- 2 cups fresh spinach, chopped
- 1 cup shredded mozzarella cheese
- 1/2 cup diced tomatoes
- 2 cloves garlic, minced
- 1 tbsp olive oil
- Salt and pepper to taste

Directions

1. Preheat the oven to 375°F (190°C).
2. In a skillet, heat the olive oil over medium heat.
3. Add the garlic and spinach, and cook until the spinach is wilted.
4. In a large bowl, combine the shredded chicken, cooked spinach, diced tomatoes, and half of the mozzarella cheese. Season with salt and pepper.
5. Stuff the bell pepper halves with the chicken mixture and place them in a baking dish.
6. Top with the remaining cheese and bake for 20-25 minutes, or until the peppers are tender and the cheese is melted.
7. Serve hot.

Ingredient Tips:

- Bell Peppers: High in vitamins A and C, and low in calories, making them great for managing blood sugar.
- Spinach: A fiber-rich vegetable that helps in blood sugar control.

Chicken and Lentil Soup

A warm and hearty soup made with chicken, lentils, and a variety of vegetables, perfect for a nutritious meal.

Servings: 2 | Prep Time: 10 mins | Cook Time: 0 mins | Carbs per serving: 8g

NUTRIENT CONTENT (PER SERVING):

- Calories: 280
- Total Fat: 6g
- Protein: 24g
- Carbohydrates: 25g
- Sugars: 6g
- Fiber: 8g
- Sodium: 400mg

Ingredients

- 2 chicken breasts, cooked and shredded
- 1 cup dried lentils, rinsed
- 1 carrot, diced
- 1 celery stalk, diced
- 1 onion, diced
- 2 cloves garlic, minced
- 4 cups chicken broth (low sodium)
- 1 tbsp olive oil
- 1 tsp cumin
- 1 tsp paprika
- Salt and pepper to taste

Directions

1. In a large pot, heat the olive oil over medium heat.
2. Add the garlic and onion and sauté until softened.
3. Add the carrot and celery and cook for a few more minutes.
4. Stir in the cumin and paprika and cook for another minute.
5. Add the lentils, chicken broth, and shredded chicken.
6. Bring to a boil, then reduce the heat and simmer for 25-30 minutes, or until the lentils are tender.
7. Season with salt and pepper to taste and serve hot.

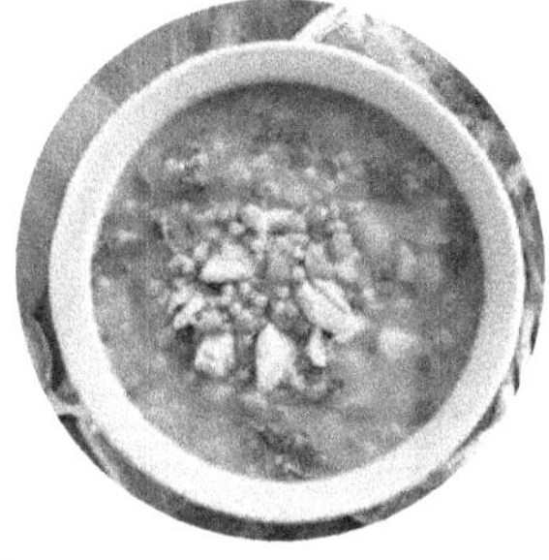

Ingredient Tips:

- Lentils: High in protein and fiber, making them excellent for managing blood sugar levels.
- Chicken Broth: Use low-sodium broth to keep the sodium content in check.

Baked Chicken with Brussels Sprouts

A simple and delicious baked chicken dish with roasted Brussels sprouts, perfect for a healthy and satisfying meal.

Servings: 4 | Prep Time: 10 mins | Cook Time: 30 mins | Carbs per Serving: 10g

NUTRIENT CONTENT (PER SERVING):

- Calories: 340
- Total Fat: 20g
- Protein: 28g
- Carbohydrates: 10g
- Sugars: 2g
- Fiber: 4g
- Sodium: 300mg

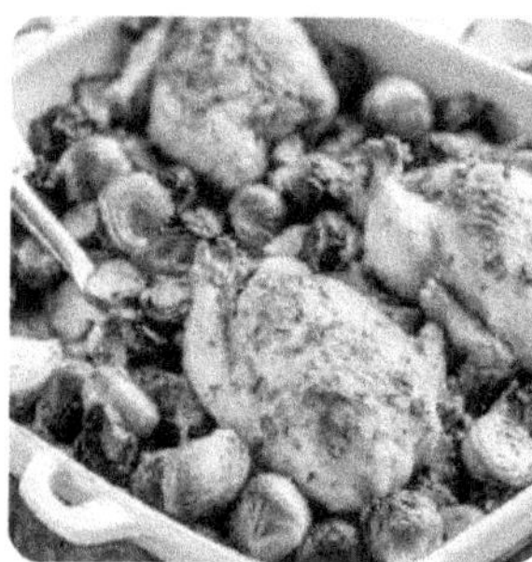

Ingredients

- 4 chicken thighs
- 2 cups Brussels sprouts, halved
- 2 tbsp olive oil
- 1 tsp garlic powder
- 1 tsp onion powder
- Salt and pepper to taste

Directions

1. Preheat the oven to 400°F (200°C).
2. In a large bowl, toss the Brussels sprouts with 1 tbsp of olive oil, garlic powder, onion powder, salt, and pepper.
3. Place the Brussels sprouts on a baking sheet.
4. Season the chicken thighs with salt and pepper and place them on top of the Brussels sprouts.
5. Drizzle the remaining olive oil over the chicken.
6. Bake for 25-30 minutes, or until the chicken is cooked through and the Brussels sprouts are tender.
7. Serve hot.

Ingredient Tips:

- Brussels Sprouts: Low in calories and high in fiber, making them a great vegetable for blood sugar control.
- Chicken Thighs: Juicier and more flavorful than chicken breasts, but still high in protein.

Chicken and Vegetable Skewers

Colorful and flavorful skewers with chicken and a variety of vegetables, perfect for grilling.

Servings: 4   Prep Time: 15 mins | Cook Time: 15 mins | Carbs per serving: 8g

NUTRIENT CONTENT (PER SERVING):

- Calories: 250
- Total Fat: 14g
- Protein: 22g
- Carbohydrates: 8g
- Sugars: 4g
- Fiber: 2g
- Sodium: 200mg

Ingredients

- 2 chicken breasts, cut into cubes
- 1 bell pepper, cut into chunks
- 1 zucchini, sliced
- 1 red onion, cut into chunks
- 1/4 cup olive oil
- 2 tbsp lemon juice
- 2 cloves garlic, minced
- Salt and pepper to taste

Directions

1. In a bowl, combine the olive oil, lemon juice, garlic, salt, and pepper.
2. Add the chicken cubes and marinate for at least 30 minutes.
3. Preheat the grill to medium-high heat.
4. Thread the chicken, bell pepper, zucchini, and red onion onto skewers.
5. Grill the skewers for 10-12 minutes, turning occasionally, until the chicken is cooked through and the vegetables are tender.
6. Serve hot.

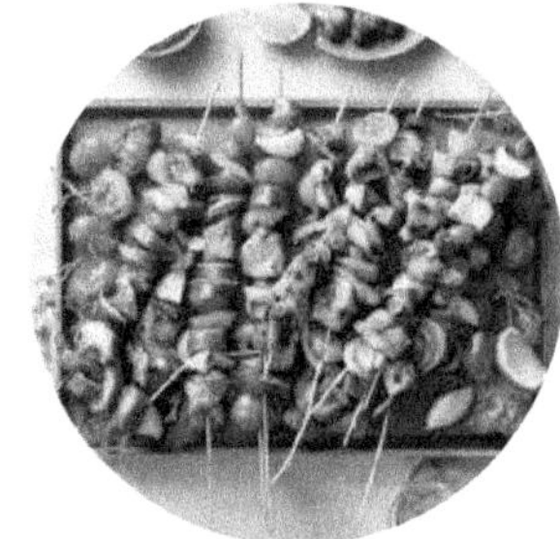

Ingredient Tips:

- Variety of Vegetables: Provides a range of vitamins and minerals, helping to manage blood sugar levels.
- Chicken Breast: Lean protein that helps keep you full and stabilize blood sugar.

Chicken Lettuce Wraps

Light and refreshing lettuce wraps filled with a flavorful chicken mixture, perfect for a quick and healthy meal.

Servings: 2 | Prep Time: 10 mins | Cook Time: 30 mins | Carbs per Serving: 12g

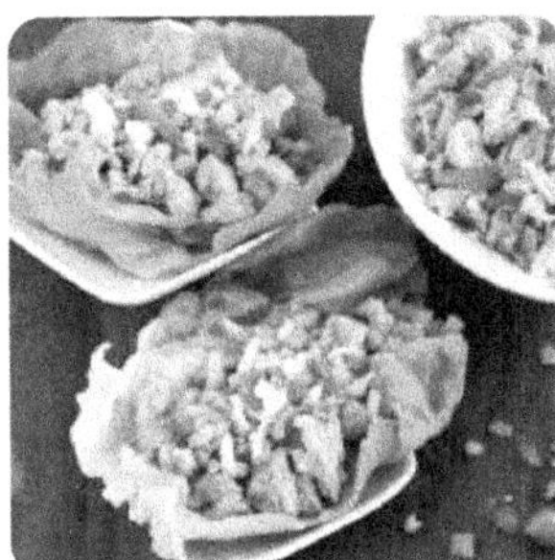

Ingredients

- 2 chicken breasts
- 1 cup cherry tomatoes, halved
- 1 cup broccoli florets
- 1 cup sliced mushrooms
- 2 tbsp olive oil
- 1/4 cup balsamic vinegar
- 1 tbsp honey (optional)
- 2 cloves garlic, minced
- Salt and pepper to taste

Directions

1. Preheat the oven to 375°F (190°C).
2. In a small bowl, whisk together the balsamic vinegar, honey (if using), garlic, salt, and pepper.
3. Place the chicken breasts in a baking dish and pour half of the balsamic mixture over them.
4. In a separate bowl, toss the vegetables with olive oil, salt, and pepper.
5. Arrange the vegetables around the chicken in the baking dish.
6. Bake for 25-30 minutes.
7. Drizzle the remaining balsamic mixture over the chicken and vegetables before serving.

Ingredient Tips:

- Balsamic Vinegar: Adds flavor without many calories, but use sparingly to keep sugar content low.
- Broccoli: High in fiber and low in calories, aiding in blood sugar control.

Turkey and Avocado Wrap

A simple and delicious turkey and avocado wrap with fresh vegetables, perfect for a quick and healthy lunch.

Servings: 4 | Prep Time: 15 mins | Cook Time: 0 mins | Carbs per serving: 20g

Ingredients

- 4 whole grain tortillas
- 1/2 lb sliced turkey breast
- 1 avocado, sliced
- 1/2 cup shredded lettuce
- 1/2 cup cherry tomatoes, halved
- 1/4 cup red onion, thinly sliced
- 2 tbsp olive oil
- 1 tbsp lime juice
- Salt and pepper to taste

Directions

1. Lay the tortillas flat on a clean surface.
2. Divide the sliced turkey breast evenly among the tortillas.
3. Top with avocado slices, shredded lettuce, cherry tomatoes, and red onion.
4. In a small bowl, whisk together the olive oil, lime juice, salt, and pepper.
5. Drizzle the dressing over the fillings.
6. Roll up the tortillas and serve.

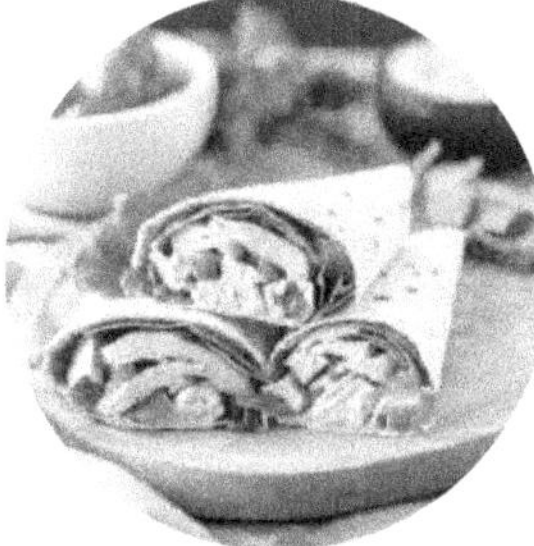

Ingredient Tips:

- Turkey Breast: Lean and high in protein, helping to keep you full and manage blood sugar levels.
- Whole Grain Tortillas: Provide complex carbohydrates and fiber, aiding in blood sugar control.

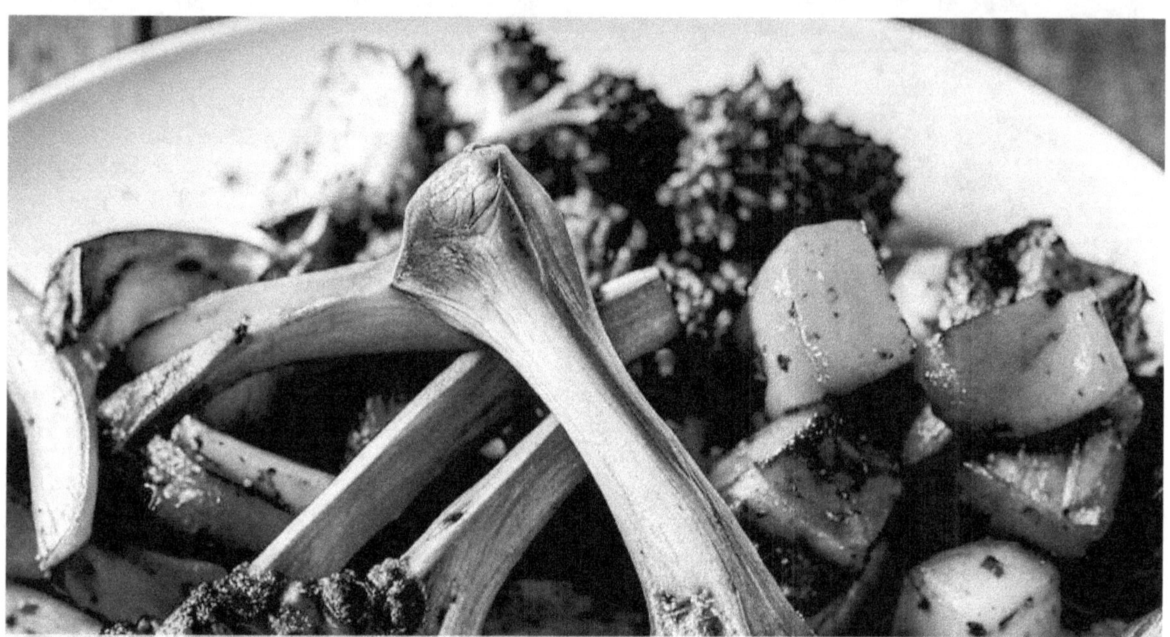

Chapter Thirteen

Beef, Pork & Lamb Recipes

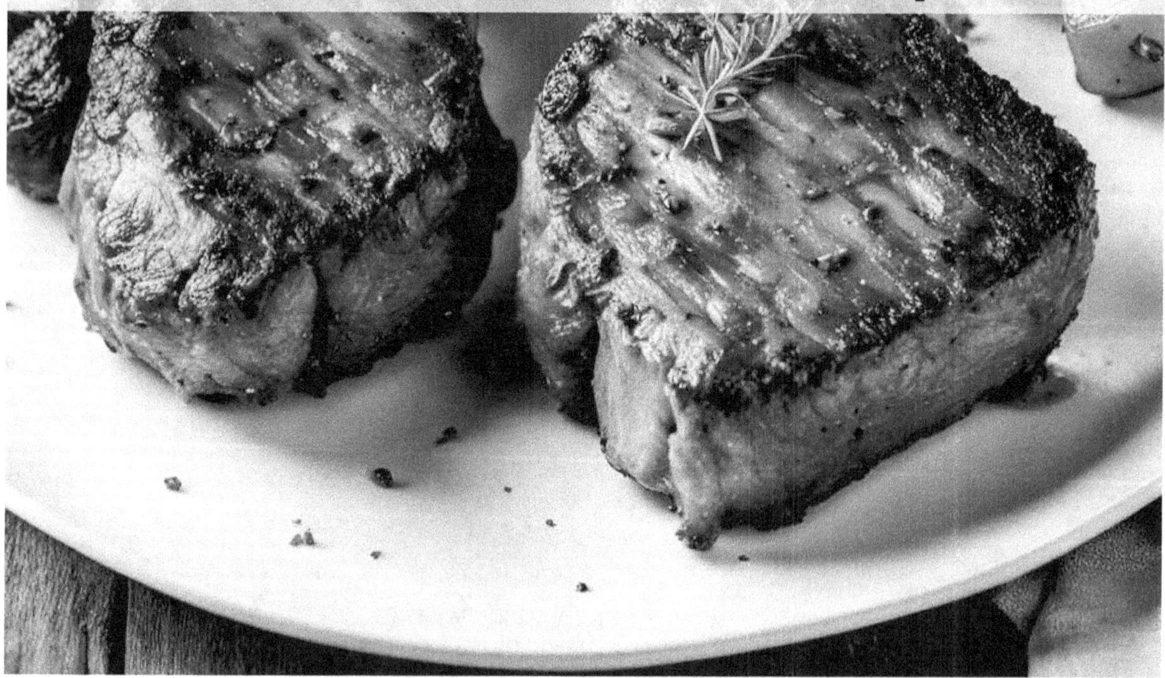

Beef and Broccoli Stir-Fry

A classic beef and broccoli stir-fry with a healthy twist, perfect for a quick and nutritious meal.

Servings: 4 | Prep Time: 10 mins | Cook Time: 15 mins | Carbs per Serving: 8g

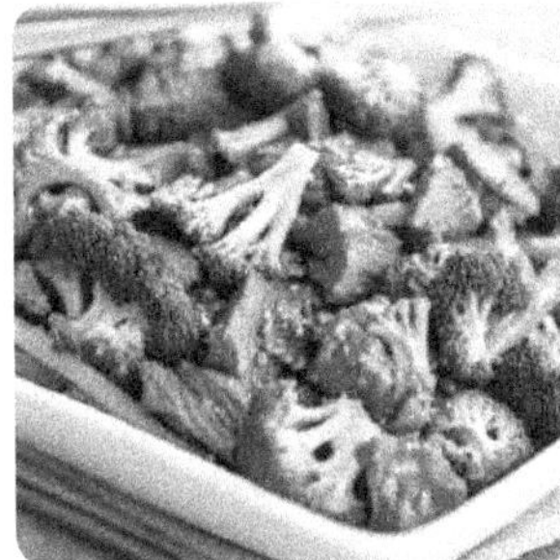

Ingredients

- 1 lb beef sirloin, thinly sliced
- 2 cups broccoli florets
- 1 bell pepper, sliced
- 1 onion, sliced
- 2 cloves garlic, minced
- 3 tbsp soy sauce (low sodium)
- 2 tbsp olive oil
- 1 tbsp sesame oil
- Salt and pepper to taste

Directions

1. In a large skillet, heat 1 tbsp of olive oil over medium-high heat.
2. Add the beef slices and cook until browned. Remove and set aside.
3. In the same skillet, heat the remaining olive oil.
4. Add the garlic and onion and sauté until softened.
5. Add the broccoli and bell pepper and cook until tender-crisp.
6. Stir in the cooked beef, soy sauce, and sesame oil.
7. Season with salt and pepper to taste and serve hot.

Ingredient Tips:

- Beef Sirloin: A lean cut of beef that is high in protein, helping to manage blood sugar levels.
- Broccoli: Low in calories and high in fiber, making it an excellent vegetable for blood sugar control.

Pork Tenderloin with Spinach

A tender and flavorful pork tenderloin served with sautéed spinach and mushrooms, perfect for a balanced meal.

Servings: 4 | Prep Time: 10 mins | Cook Time: 25 mins | Carbs per serving: 6g

Ingredients

- 1 lb pork tenderloin
- 2 cups spinach
- 1 cup mushrooms, sliced
- 2 cloves garlic, minced
- 2 tbsp olive oil
- 1 tsp dried thyme
- Salt and pepper to taste

Directions

1. Preheat the oven to 375°F (190°C).
2. Season the pork tenderloin with thyme, salt, & pepper.
3. In an oven-safe skillet, heat 1 tbsp of olive oil over medium-high heat.
4. Sear the pork tenderloin on all sides.
5. Transfer the skillet to the oven and roast for 20-25 minutes, or until the internal temperature reaches 145°F (63°C). Let rest before slicing.
6. In a separate skillet, heat the remaining olive oil over medium heat.
7. Add the garlic and sauté until fragrant.
8. Add the mushrooms and cook until softened.
9. Add the spinach and cook until wilted. Season with salt and pepper to taste.
10. Serve hot

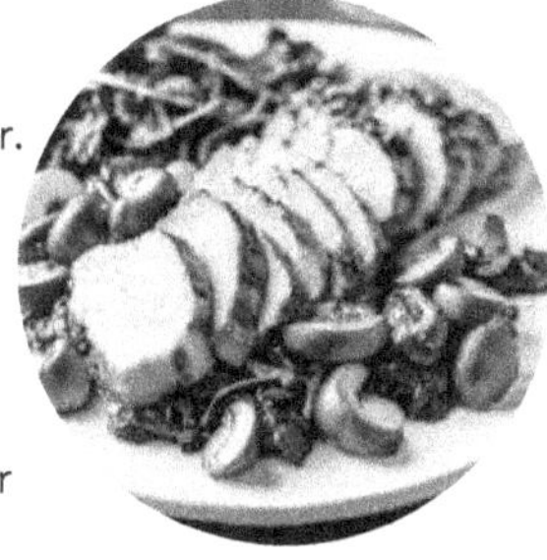

Ingredient Tips:

- Pork Tenderloin: A lean source of protein that helps keep you full and manage blood sugar levels.
- Spinach: High in fiber and nutrients, making it a great addition to any meal.

Lamb Chops with Roasted Vegetables

Succulent lamb chops served with a side of roasted vegetables for a hearty and nutritious meal.

Servings: 4 | Prep Time: 10 mins | Cook Time: 25 mins | Carbs per Serving: 10g

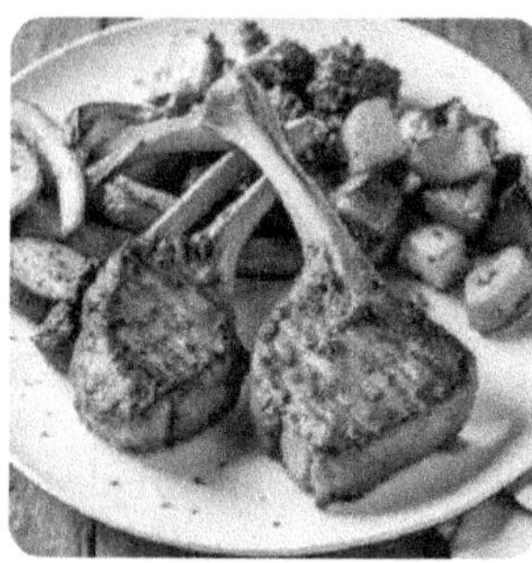

Ingredients

- 4 lamb chops
- 2 cups mixed vegetables (carrots, bell peppers, zucchini)
- 2 cloves garlic, minced
- 3 tbsp olive oil
- 1 tbsp fresh rosemary, chopped
- Salt and pepper to taste

Directions

1. Preheat the oven to 400°F (200°C).
2. In a large bowl, toss the mixed vegetables with 2 tbsp of olive oil, garlic, rosemary, salt, and pepper.
3. Spread the vegetables on a baking sheet and roast for 20-25 minutes, or until tender and slightly caramelized.
4. Meanwhile, heat the remaining olive oil in a skillet over medium-high heat.
5. Season the lamb chops with salt and pepper.
6. Sear the lamb chops for 3-4 minutes on each side.
7. Let the lamb chops rest for a few minutes before serving with the roasted vegetables.

Ingredient Tips:

- Lamb Chops: High in protein and healthy fats, making them a satisfying choice for managing blood sugar levels.
- Mixed Vegetables: Provide a variety of nutrients and fiber, aiding in blood sugar control.

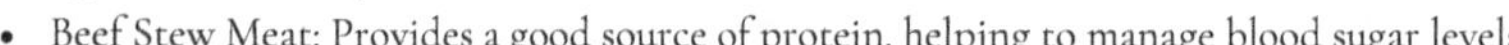

Beef and Lentil Stew

A hearty and nutritious beef and lentil stew, perfect for a filling and balanced meal.

Servings: 4   Prep Time: 10 mins | Cook Time: 35 mins | Carbs per serving: 25g

Ingredients

- 1 lb beef stew meat, cubed
- 1 cup lentils, rinsed
- 1 cup diced tomatoes
- 2 carrots, diced
- 1 onion, diced
- 2 cloves garlic, minced
- 4 cups beef broth (low sodium)
- 2 tbsp olive oil
- 1 tsp cumin
- 1 tsp paprika
- Salt and pepper to taste

Directions

1. In a large pot, heat the olive oil over medium heat.
2. Add the beef and cook until browned on all sides. Remove and set aside.
3. In the same pot, add the garlic and onion and sauté until softened.
4. Add the carrots and cook for a few minutes.
5. Stir in the cumin and paprika and cook for another minute.
6. Add the lentils, diced tomatoes, beef broth, and browned beef.
7. Bring to a boil, then reduce the heat and simmer for 30-35 minutes, or until the lentils are tender.
8. Season with salt and pepper to taste and serve hot.

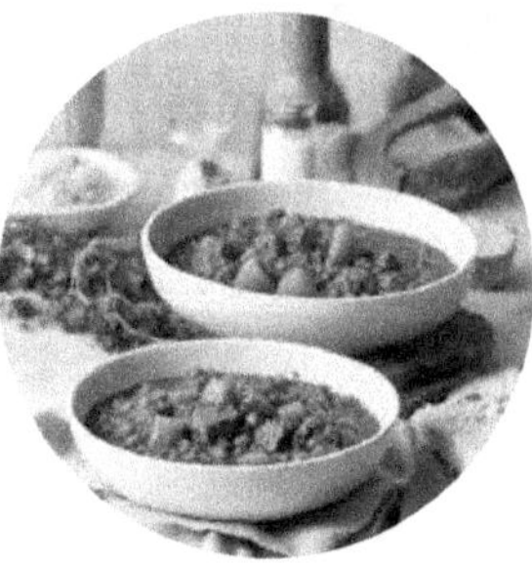

Ingredient Tips:

- Beef Stew Meat: Provides a good source of protein, helping to manage blood sugar levels.
- Lentils: High in protein and fiber, making them excellent for blood sugar control.

Lamb and Quinoa Salad

A hearty and nutritious lamb and quinoa salad with fresh vegetables, perfect for a balanced and satisfying meal.

Servings: 4 | Prep Time: 10 mins | Cook Time: 25 mins | Carbs per Serving: 10g

NUTRIENT CONTENT (PER SERVING):

- Calories: 350
- Total Fat: 18g
- Protein: 24g
- Carbohydrates: 20g
- Sugars: 4g
- Fiber: 4g
- Sodium: 300mg

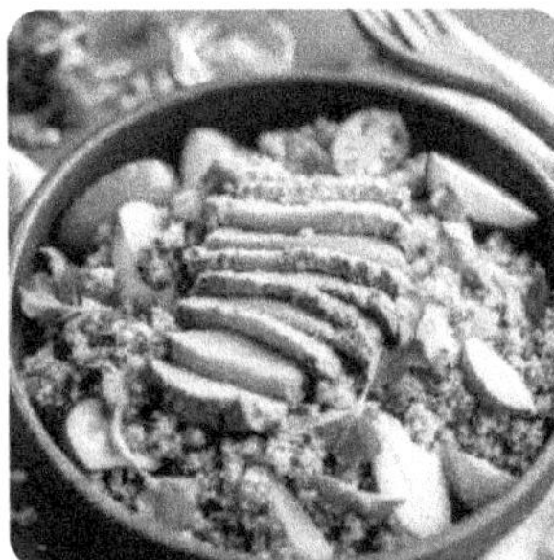

Ingredients

- 1 lb lamb, cooked and cubed
- 1 cup quinoa, cooked
- 1 cup cherry tomatoes, halved
- 1 cucumber, diced
- 1/4 cup red onion, diced
- 2 tbsp olive oil
- 1 tbsp lemon juice
- Salt and pepper to taste

Directions

1. In a large bowl, combine the cooked lamb, quinoa, cherry tomatoes, cucumber, and red onion.
2. In a small bowl, whisk together the olive oil, lemon juice, salt, and pepper.
3. Pour the dressing over the salad and toss to combine.
4. Serve immediately.

Ingredient Tips:

- Lamb: High in protein and healthy fats, making it a satisfying choice for managing blood sugar levels.
- Quinoa: A whole grain that is high in protein and fiber, aiding in blood sugar control.

Beef and Cauliflower Rice Bowl

A low-carb beef and cauliflower rice bowl with fresh vegetables, perfect for a quick and healthy meal.

Servings: 4   Prep Time: 10 mins | Cook Time: 35 mins | Carbs per serving: 25g

NUTRIENT CONTENT (PER SERVING):

- Calories: 280
- Total Fat: 16g
- Protein: 24g
- Carbohydrates: 8g
- Sugars: 4g
- Fiber: 4g
- Sodium: 400mg

Ingredients

- 1 lb ground beef (lean)
- 2 cups cauliflower rice
- 1 cup bell pepper, diced
- 1 cup spinach
- 2 cloves garlic, minced
- 2 tbsp olive oil
- 1 tbsp soy sauce (low sodium)
- Salt and pepper to taste

Directions

1. In a large skillet, heat the olive oil over medium heat.
2. Add the garlic and cook until fragrant.
3. Add the ground beef and cook until browned.
4. Stir in the bell pepper and cook until tender.
5. Add the cauliflower rice and cook until heated through.
6. Stir in the spinach and soy sauce and cook until wilted.
7. Season with salt and pepper to taste and serve hot.

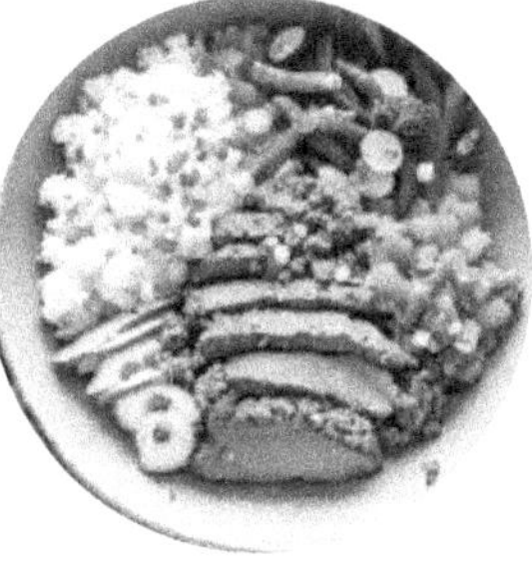

Ingredient Tips:

- Ground Beef: A lean source of protein that helps keep you full and manage blood sugar levels.
- Cauliflower Rice: A low-carb alternative to rice, helping to keep carbohydrate intake low.

Pork and Cabbage Stir-Fry

: A quick and easy pork stir-fry with cabbage and a flavorful sauce, perfect for a healthy and satisfying meal.

Servings: 4 | Prep Time: 10 mins | Cook Time: 15 mins | Carbs per Serving: 10g

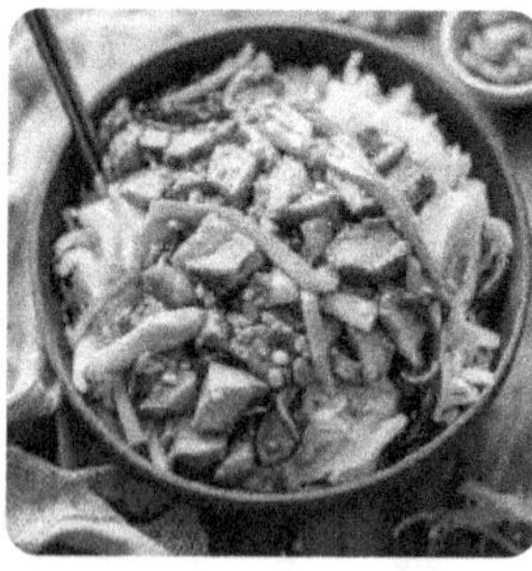

Ingredients

- 1 lb pork loin, thinly sliced
- 4 cups shredded cabbage
- 1 bell pepper, sliced
- 2 cloves garlic, minced
- 2 tbsp soy sauce (low sodium)
- 2 tbsp olive oil
- 1 tsp sesame oil
- Salt and pepper to taste

Directions

1. In a large skillet, heat 1 tbsp of olive oil over medium-high heat.
2. Add the pork slices and cook until browned. Remove and set aside.
3. In the same skillet, heat the remaining olive oil.
4. Add the garlic and sauté until fragrant.
5. Add the cabbage and bell pepper and cook until tender-crisp.
6. Stir in the cooked pork, soy sauce, and sesame oil.
7. Season with salt and pepper to taste and serve hot.

Ingredient Tips:

- Pork Loin: A lean source of protein that helps keep you full and manage blood sugar levels.
- Cabbage: Low in calories and high in fiber, making it a great vegetable for blood sugar control.

Lamb and Vegetable Kebabs

Flavorful lamb and vegetable kebabs, perfect for grilling and enjoying a balanced meal.

Servings: 4 | Prep Time: 15 mins | Cook Time: 12 mins | Carbs per serving: 8g

Ingredients

- 1 lb lamb, cubed
- 1 zucchini, sliced
- 1 bell pepper, cubed
- 1 red onion, cubed
- 2 tbsp olive oil
- 1 tbsp lemon juice
- 1 tsp dried oregano
- Salt and pepper to taste.

Directions

1. In a large bowl, combine the olive oil, lemon juice, oregano, salt, and pepper.
2. Add the lamb and vegetables to the bowl and toss to coat.
3. Thread the lamb and vegetables onto skewers.
4. Grill the kebabs over medium-high heat for 10-12 minutes, turning occasionally, until the lamb is cooked to your desired level of doneness.
5. Serve hot.

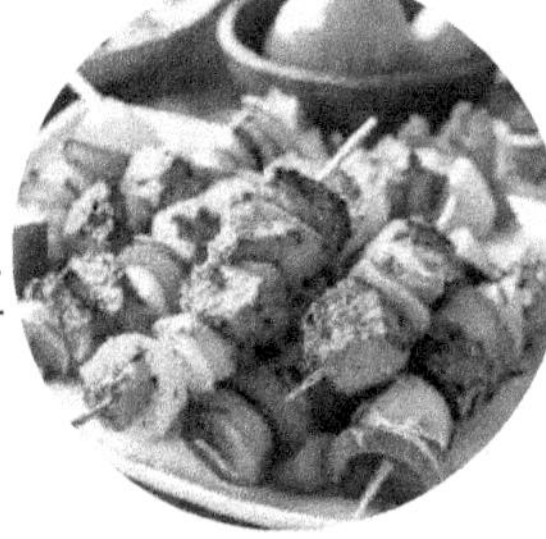

Ingredient Tips:

- Lamb: High in protein and healthy fats, making it a satisfying choice for managing blood sugar levels.
- Vegetables: Provide a variety of nutrients and fiber, aiding in blood sugar control.

Beef and Apple Skillet

A savory beef and apple skillet dish with a hint of sweetness from the apples, perfect for a balanced and delicious meal.

Servings: 4 | Prep Time: 10 mins | Cook Time: 15 mins | Carbs per Serving: 6g

NUTRIENT CONTENT (PER SERVING):

- Calories: 280
- Total Fat: 18g
- Protein: 24g
- Carbohydrates: 6g
- Sugars: 4g
- Fiber: 2g
- Sodium: 350mg

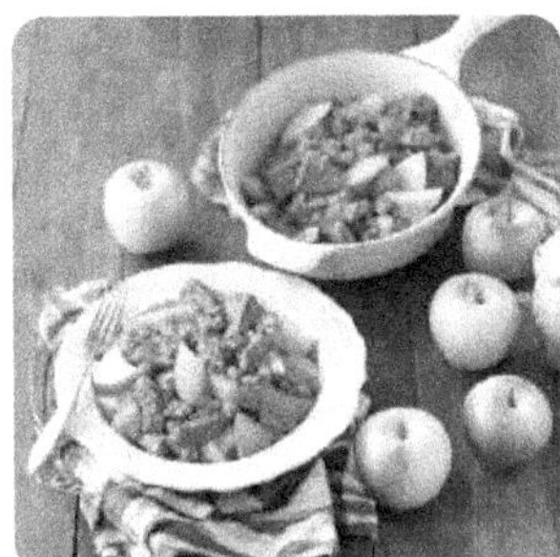

Ingredients

- 1 lb ground beef (lean)
- 2 cups diced tomatoes
- 1 onion, diced
- 2 cloves garlic, minced
- 2 tbsp olive oil
- 1 tsp dried basil
- 1 tsp dried oregano
- Salt and pepper to taste

Directions

1. In a large skillet, heat the olive oil over medium heat.
2. Add the garlic and onion and sauté until softened.
3. Add the ground beef and cook until browned.
4. Stir in the diced tomatoes, basil, oregano, salt, and pepper.
5. Simmer for 10-15 minutes, or until the flavors are well combined.
6. Serve hot.

Ingredient Tips:

- Ground Beef: A lean source of protein that helps keep you full and manage blood sugar levels.
- Tomatoes: Low in calories and high in nutrients, making them a great addition to any meal.

Pork and Apple Skillet

A savory pork and apple skillet dish with a hint of sweetness from the apples, perfect for a balanced and delicious meal.

Servings: 4 | Prep Time: 10 mins | Cook Time: 15 mins | Carbs per serving: 12g

NUTRIENT CONTENT (PER SERVING):

- Calories: 300
- Total Fat: 16g
- Protein: 26g
- Carbohydrates: 12g
- Sugars: 8g
- Fiber: 2g
- Sodium: 350mg

Ingredients

- 1 lb pork chops
- 2 apples, sliced
- 1 onion, sliced
- 2 cloves garlic, minced
- 2 tbsp olive oil
- 1 tsp dried thyme
- Salt and pepper to taste

Directions

1. Season the pork chops with salt, pepper, and thyme.
2. In a large skillet, heat the olive oil over medium-high heat.
3. Add the pork chops and cook until browned on both sides. Remove and set aside.
4. In the same skillet, add the garlic and onion and sauté until softened.
5. Add the apple slices and cook until tender.
6. Return the pork chops to the skillet and cook until heated through.
7. Serve hot.

Ingredient Tips:

- Pork Chops: A lean source of protein that helps keep you full and manage blood sugar levels.
- Apples: Provide a natural sweetness and fiber, helping to manage blood sugar levels.

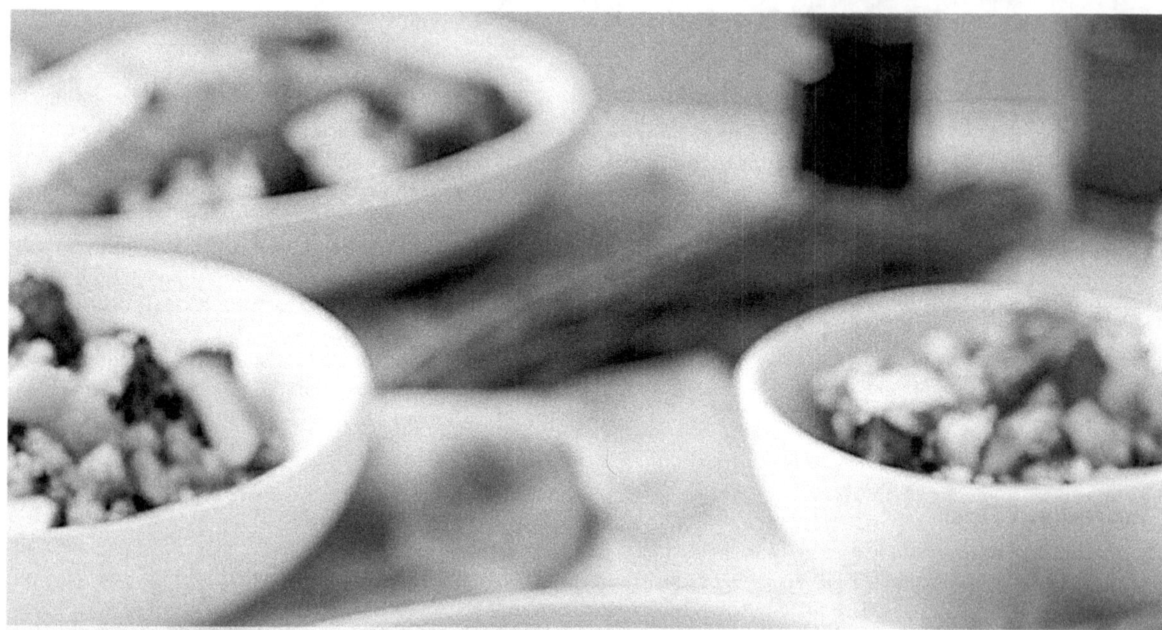

Chapter Fourteen

Fish and Seafood Recipes

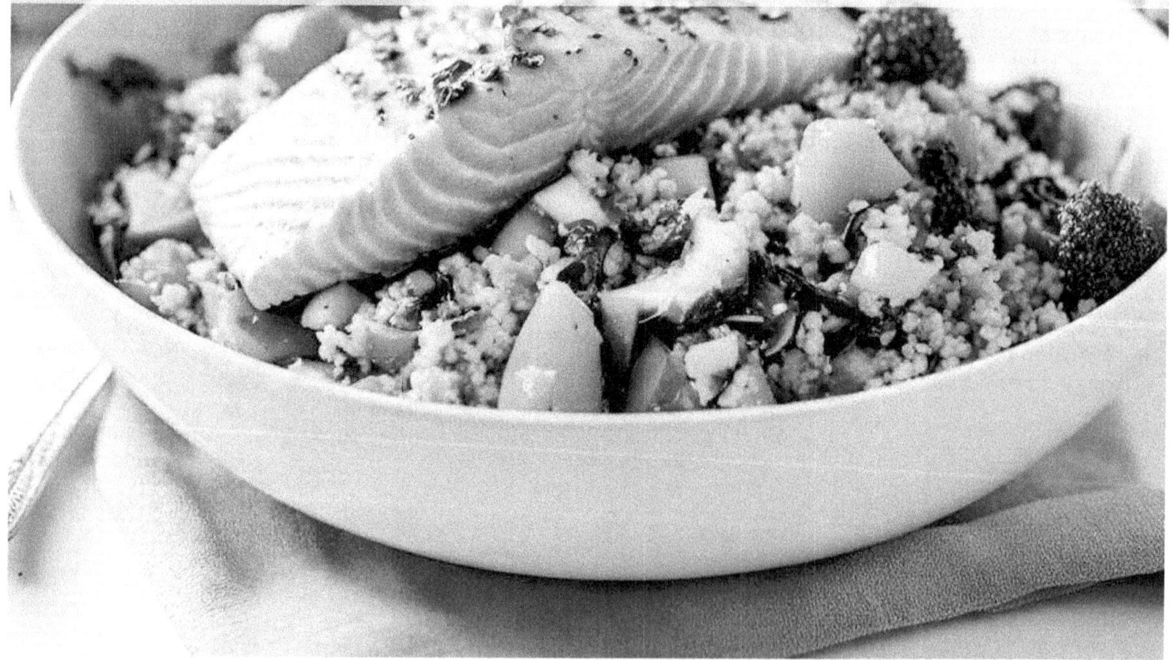

Grilled Salmon with Avocado Salsa

A simple yet flavorful dish with grilled salmon topped with a refreshing avocado salsa. Perfect for a nutritious and satisfying meal.

Servings: 2 | Prep Time: 10 mins | Cook Time: 10 mins | Carbs per Serving: 8g

NUTRIENT CONTENT (PER SERVING):

- Calories: 360
- Total Fat: 25g
- Protein: 28g
- Carbohydrates: 8g
- Sugars: 2g
- Fiber: 6g
- Sodium: 120mg

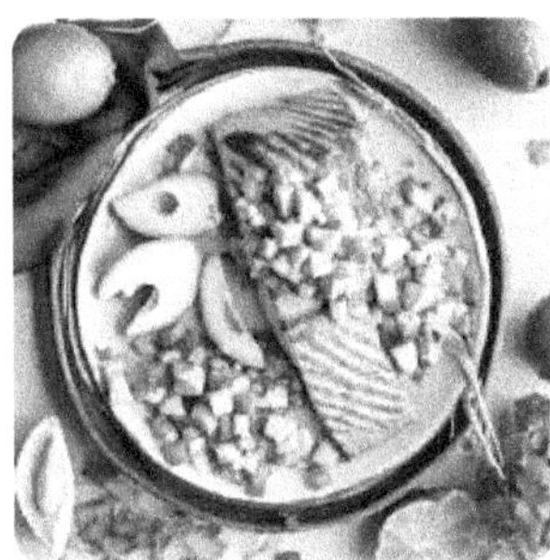

Ingredients

- 2 salmon fillets
- 1 avocado, diced
- 1 small red onion, finely chopped
- 1 tomato, diced
- 1 tbsp olive oil
- 1 tbsp lime juice
- Salt and pepper to taste
- Fresh cilantro for garnish

Directions

1. Preheat the grill to medium-high heat.
2. Season the salmon fillets with salt and pepper.
3. Grill the salmon for about 4-5 minutes per side, or until cooked through.
4. In a bowl, combine the diced avocado, red onion, tomato, olive oil, lime juice, salt, and pepper.
5. Top the grilled salmon with the avocado salsa and garnish with fresh cilantro before serving.

Ingredient Tips:

- Salmon: High in omega-3 fatty acids, which help reduce inflammation and improve blood sugar control.
- Avocado: Provides healthy fats and fiber, aiding in blood sugar management.

Shrimp and Vegetable Stir-Fry

A quick and easy shrimp stir-fry with a variety of fresh vegetables, perfect for a light and balanced meal.

Servings: 4   Prep Time: 10 mins | Cook Time: 10 mins | Carbs per serving: 8g

NUTRIENT CONTENT (PER SERVING):

- Calories: 200
- Total Fat: 12g
- Protein: 20g
- Carbohydrates: 8g
- Sugars: 4g
- Fiber: 2g
- Sodium: 300mg

Ingredients

- 1 lb shrimp, peeled and deveined
- 1 bell pepper, sliced
- 1 zucchini, sliced
- 1 cup snap peas
- 2 cloves garlic, minced
- 2 tbsp olive oil
- 2 tbsp low-sodium soy sauce
- 1 tbsp sesame oil
- Salt and pepper to taste

Directions

1. In a large skillet, heat 1 tbsp of olive oil over medium-high heat.
2. Add the shrimp and cook until pink and opaque. Remove and set aside.
3. In the same skillet, heat the remaining olive oil.
4. Add the garlic and sauté until fragrant.
5. Add the bell pepper, zucchini, and snap peas and cook until tender-crisp.
6. Stir in the cooked shrimp, soy sauce, and sesame oil.
7. Season with salt and pepper to taste and serve hot.

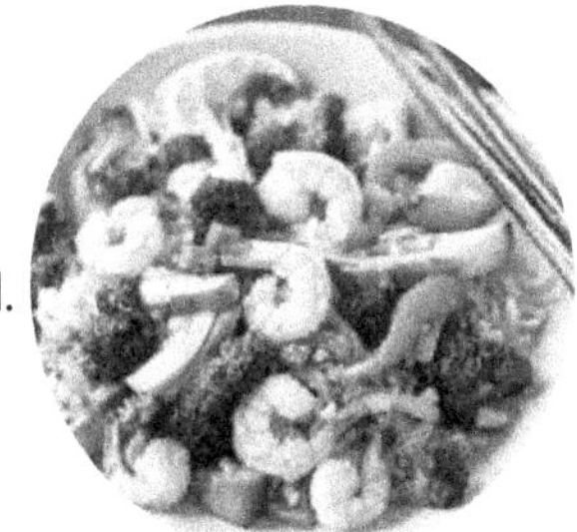

Ingredient Tips:

- Shrimp: Low in calories and high in protein, making them a great choice for blood sugar management.
- Snap Peas: Low in calories and high in fiber, helping to control blood sugar levels.

Baked Cod with Spinach & Tomatoes

A light and healthy baked cod dish with a bed of spinach and cherry tomatoes. Perfect for a nutritious and satisfying meal.

Servings: 2 | Prep Time: 10 mins | Cook Time:1 0 mins | Carbs per Serving: 6g

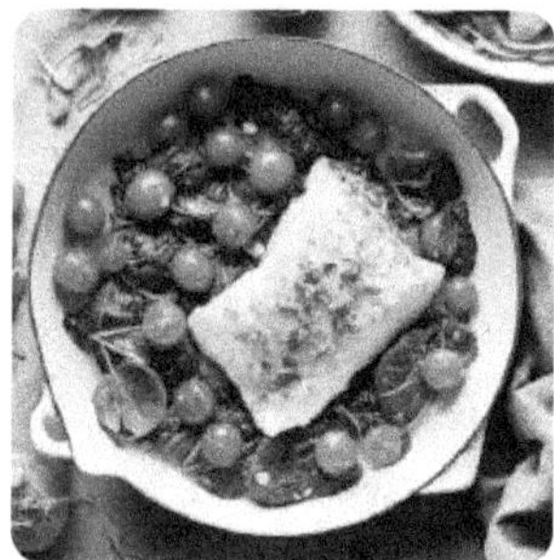

Ingredients

- 2 cod fillets
- 2 cups fresh spinach
- 1 cup cherry tomatoes, halved
- 1 clove garlic, minced
- 2 tbsp olive oil
- 1 tbsp lemon juice
- Salt and pepper to taste

Directions

1. Preheat the oven to 400°F (200°C).
2. Place the cod fillets on a baking sheet lined with parchment paper.
3. Drizzle with olive oil and lemon juice, and season with salt and pepper.
4. In a bowl, toss the spinach, cherry tomatoes, and garlic with a little olive oil.
5. Arrange the spinach and tomato mixture around the cod fillets.
6. Bake for 15-20 minutes, or until the cod is cooked through and flakes easily with a fork.

Ingredient Tips:

- Cod: A lean source of protein that helps keep you full and manage blood sugar levels.
- Spinach: Low in calories and high in fiber and nutrients, making it a great vegetable for blood sugar control.

Tuna and Avocado Salad

A simple and delicious tuna salad with creamy avocado and fresh vegetables, perfect for a quick and healthy lunch.

Servings: 2 | Prep Time: 10 mins | Cook Time: 0 mins | Carbs per serving: 8g

Ingredients

- 1 can tuna in water, drained
- 1 avocado, diced
- 1/2 cup cherry tomatoes, halved
- 1/4 cup red onion, diced
- 2 tbsp olive oil
- 1 tbsp lemon juice
- Salt and pepper to taste

Directions

1. In a large bowl, combine the tuna, avocado, cherry tomatoes, and red onion.
2. In a small bowl, whisk together the olive oil, lemon juice, salt, and pepper.
3. Pour the dressing over the tuna mixture and toss to combine.
4. Serve immediately.

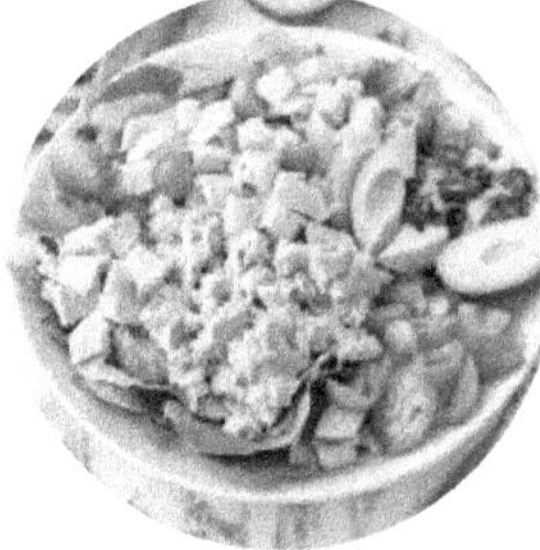

Ingredient Tips:

- Tuna: High in protein and omega-3 fatty acids, helping to manage blood sugar levels and promote heart health.
- Avocado: Provides healthy fats and fiber, aiding in blood sugar control.

Garlic Butter Shrimp and Asparagus

A quick and delicious garlic butter shrimp dish with tender asparagus. Perfect for a light and flavorful meal.

Servings: 2 | Prep Time: 10 mins | Cook Time:1 0 mins | Carbs per Serving: 6g

NUTRIENT CONTENT (PER SERVING):

- Calories: 200
- Total Fat: 12g
- Protein: 20g
- Carbohydrates: 6g
- Sugars: 2g
- Fiber: 2g
- Sodium: 350mg

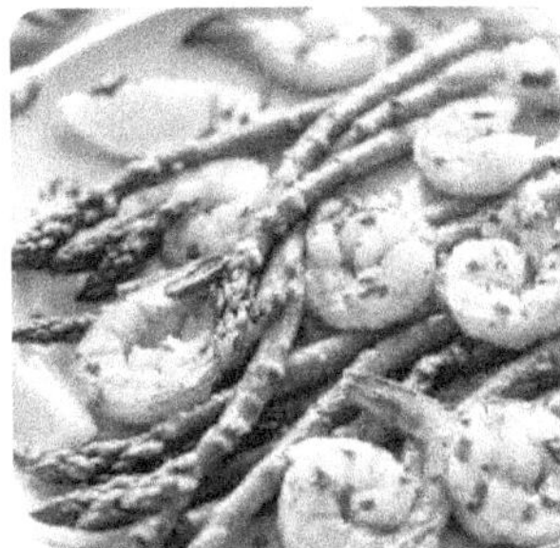

Ingredients

- 1 lb shrimp, peeled and deveined
- 1 bunch asparagus, trimmed and cut into bite-sized pieces
- 3 cloves garlic, minced
- 2 tbsp butter
- 1 tbsp olive oil
- Salt and pepper to taste
- Lemon wedges for serving

Directions

1. In a large skillet, heat the olive oil and butter over medium heat.
2. Add the garlic and sauté until fragrant.
3. Add the shrimp and cook until pink and opaque, about 2-3 minutes per side.
4. Add the asparagus and cook until tender-crisp, about 3-4 minutes.
5. Season with salt and pepper to taste and serve with lemon wedges.

Ingredient Tips:

- Shrimp: Low in calories and high in protein, making them a great choice for blood sugar management.
- Asparagus: Low in calories and high in fiber, helping to control blood sugar levels.

Seared Scallops with Spinach and Mushrooms

A sophisticated dish with seared scallops served on a bed of sautéed spinach and mushrooms. Perfect for a special meal.

Servings: 4 | Prep Time: 10 mins | Cook Time: 10 mins | Carbs per serving: 8g

NUTRIENT CONTENT (PER SERVING):

- Calories: 250
- Total Fat: 18g
- Protein: 16g
- Carbohydrates: 8g
- Sugars: 4g
- Fiber: 2g
- Sodium: 300mg

Ingredients

- 1 lb scallops
- 2 cups fresh spinach
- 1 cup sliced mushrooms
- 2 cloves garlic, minced
- 2 tbsp olive oil
- 1 tbsp butter
- Salt and pepper to taste

Directions

1. In a large skillet, heat the olive oil and butter over medium-high heat.
2. Season the scallops with salt and pepper.
3. Sear the scallops for about 2-3 minutes per side, until golden brown and cooked through. Remove and set aside.
4. In the same skillet, add the garlic and sauté until fragrant.
5. Add the mushrooms and cook until tender.
6. Add the spinach and cook until wilted.
7. Season with salt and pepper to taste and serve with the seared scallops.

Ingredient Tips:

- Scallops: High in protein and low in fat, making them a great option for blood sugar management.
- Spinach: Low in calories and high in fiber and nutrients, aiding in blood sugar control.

Lemon Herb Baked Tilapia

A light and refreshing lemon herb baked tilapia, perfect for a healthy and delicious meal.

Servings: 4 | Prep Time: 10 mins | Cook Time: 20 mins | Carbs per Serving: 6g

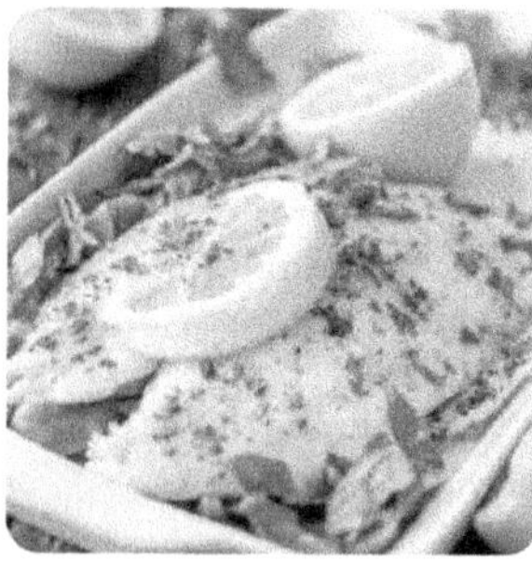

Ingredients

- 4 tilapia fillets
- 2 tbsp olive oil
- 1 lemon, sliced
- 2 cloves garlic, minced
- 1 tbsp fresh parsley, chopped
- 1 tbsp fresh dill, chopped
- Salt and pepper to taste

Directions

1. Preheat the oven to 375°F (190°C).
2. Place the tilapia fillets on a baking sheet lined with parchment paper.
3. Drizzle with olive oil and sprinkle with garlic, parsley, dill, salt, and pepper.
4. Top with lemon slices.
5. Bake for 15-20 minutes, or until the fish flakes easily with a fork.

Ingredient Tips:

- Tilapia: Low in calories and high in protein, making them a great choice for blood sugar management.
- Lemon: Low in calories and high in fiber, helping to control blood sugar levels.

Salmon and Quinoa Salad

A nutritious and filling salmon and quinoa salad with fresh vegetables, perfect for a balanced and satisfying meal.

Servings: 2 | Prep Time: 15 mins | Cook Time: 10 mins | Carbs per serving: 22g

Ingredients

- 2 salmon fillets
- 1 cup cooked quinoa
- 1 cup cherry tomatoes, halved
- 1 cucumber, diced
- 1/4 cup red onion, diced
- 2 tbsp olive oil
- 1 tbsp lemon juice
- Salt and pepper to taste
- Fresh parsley for garnish

Directions

1. Preheat the grill to medium-high heat.
2. Season the salmon fillets with salt and pepper.
3. Grill the salmon for about 4-5 minutes per side, or until cooked through. Let rest, then flake into pieces.
4. In a large bowl, combine the cooked quinoa, cherry tomatoes, cucumber, and red onion.
5. In a small bowl, whisk together the olive oil, lemon juice, salt, and pepper.
6. Pour the dressing over the quinoa mixture and toss to combine.
7. Top with flaked salmon and garnish with fresh parsley before serving.

Ingredient Tips:

- Salmon: High in omega-3 fatty acids, which help reduce inflammation and improve blood sugar control.
- Quinoa: A whole grain that provides protein and fiber, aiding in blood sugar management.

Spicy Shrimp with Cauliflower Rice

A flavorful and low-carb dish with spicy garlic shrimp served over cauliflower rice. Perfect for a light and healthy meal.

NUTRIENT CONTENT (PER SERVING):

- Calories: 180
- Total Fat: 10g
- Protein: 20g
- Carbohydrates: 2g
- Sugars: 2g
- Fiber: 2g
- Sodium: 350mg

Servings: 4 | Prep Time: 10 mins | Cook Time: 15 mins | Carbs per Serving: 6g

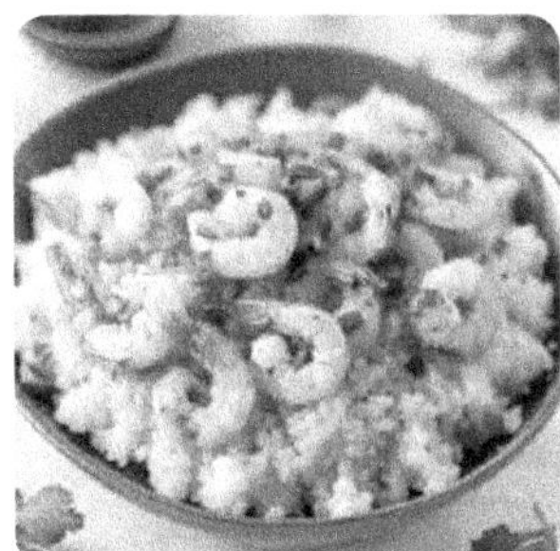

Ingredients

- 1 lb shrimp, peeled and deveined
- 3 cups cauliflower rice
- 3 cloves garlic, minced
- 1 tbsp olive oil
- 1 tbsp butter
- 1 tsp paprika
- 1/2 tsp red pepper flakes
- Salt and pepper to taste
- Fresh parsley for garnish

Directions

1. In a large skillet, heat the olive oil and butter over medium heat.
2. Add the garlic and sauté until fragrant.
3. Add the shrimp, paprika, red pepper flakes, salt, and pepper.
4. Cook until the shrimp are pink and opaque, about 2-3 minutes per side. Remove and set aside.
5. In the same skillet, add the cauliflower rice and cook until tender, about 5-7 minutes.
6. Season the cauliflower rice with salt and pepper to taste.
7. Serve the shrimp over the cauliflower rice and garnish with fresh parsley.

Ingredient Tips:

- Shrimps: Low in calories and high in protein, making them a great choice for blood sugar management.
- Cauliflower Rice: Low in calories and high in fiber, helping to control blood sugar levels.

Lemon Garlic Butter Fish

A simple and delicious lemon garlic butter fish, perfect for a quick and healthy meal.

NUTRIENT CONTENT (PER SERVING):

- Calories: 180
- Total Fat: 10g
- Protein: 20g
- Carbohydrates: 2g
- Sugars: 4g
- Fiber: 2g
- Sodium: 300mg

Servings: 4 | Prep Time: 10 mins | Cook Time: 20 mins | Carbs per serving: 2g

Ingredients

- 4 white fish fillets (such as cod or haddock)
- 3 cloves garlic, minced
- 3 tbsp butter
- 1 lemon, juiced
- Salt and pepper to taste
- Fresh parsley for garnish

Directions

1. Preheat the oven to 375°F (190°C).
2. Place the fish fillets on a baking sheet lined with parchment paper.
3. In a small saucepan, melt the butter over medium heat.
4. Add the garlic and cook until fragrant.
5. Remove from heat and stir in the lemon juice.
6. Pour the lemon garlic butter over the fish fillets.
7. Season with salt and pepper to taste.
8. Bake for 15-20 minutes, or until the fish flakes easily with a fork.
9. Garnish with fresh parsley before serving.

Ingredient Tips:

- White Fish: A lean source of protein that helps keep you full and manage blood sugar levels.
- Garlic: Adds flavor without adding calories or carbohydrates.

Chapter Fifteen

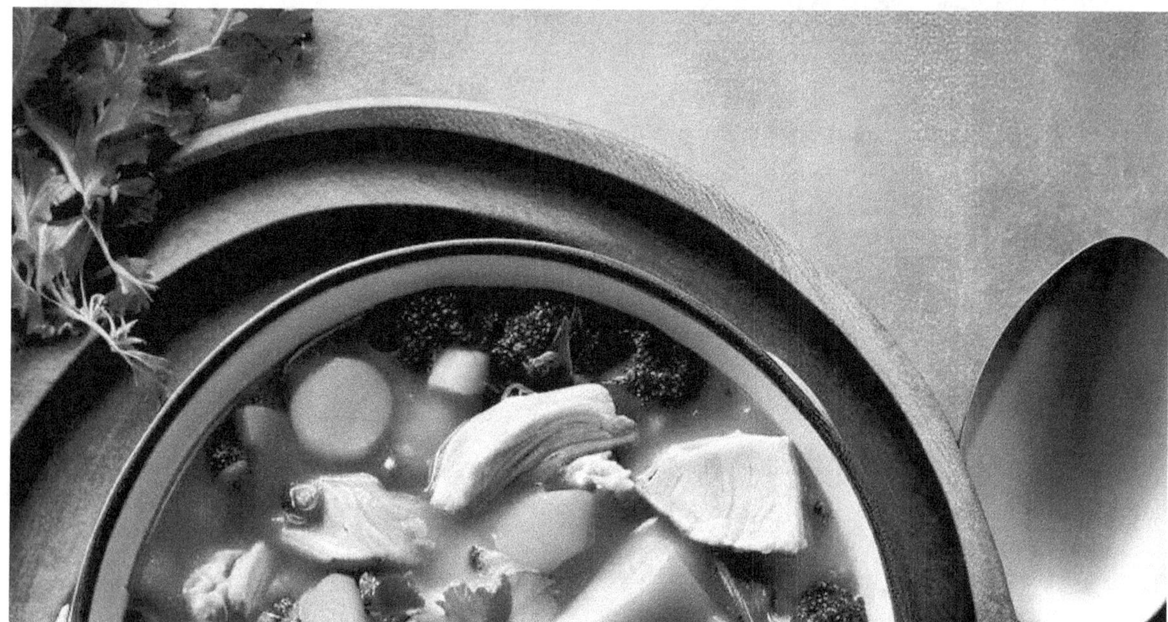

Soup Recipes

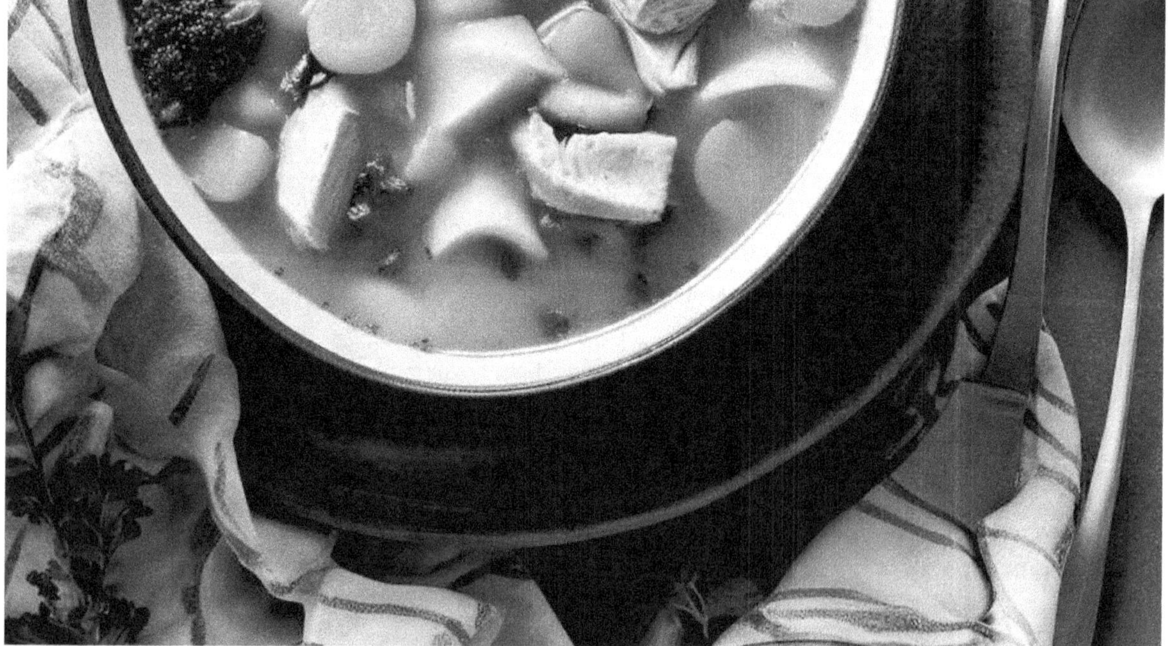

Chicken and Vegetable Soup

A hearty and nutritious soup with lean chicken and a variety of vegetables, perfect for a satisfying and balanced meal.

Servings: 4 | Prep Time: 10 mins | Cook Time: 30 mins | Carbs per Serving: 8g

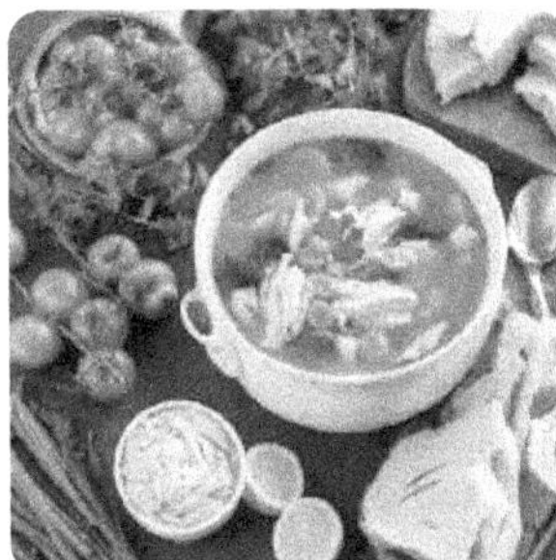

Ingredients

- 2 chicken breasts, diced
- 1 onion, diced
- 2 carrots, sliced
- 2 celery stalks, sliced
- 1 cup spinach
- 2 cloves garlic, minced
- 4 cups low-sodium chicken broth
- 1 tbsp olive oil
- Salt and pepper to taste.

Directions

1. In a large pot, heat the olive oil over medium heat.
2. Add the garlic and onion and sauté until softened.
3. Add the carrots and celery and cook for a few more minutes.
4. Add the diced chicken and cook until browned.
5. Pour in the chicken broth and bring to a boil.
6. Reduce heat and simmer for 20 minutes.
7. Add the spinach and cook for another 5 minutes.
8. Season with salt and pepper to taste and serve hot.

Ingredient Tips:

- Chicken Breast: Lean and high in protein, helping to keep you full and manage blood sugar levels.
- Spinach: Low in calories and high in fiber, making it great for blood sugar control.

Lentil and Spinach Soup

A flavorful and protein-packed lentil soup with spinach and spices, ideal for a nutritious lunch or dinner.

Servings: 4   Prep Time: 10 mins | Cook Time: 30 mins | Carbs per serving: 25g

Ingredients

- 1 cup dried lentils, rinsed
- 1 onion, diced
- 2 cloves garlic, minced
- 1 carrot, diced
- 2 cups spinach
- 4 cups vegetable broth (low sodium)
- 1 tbsp olive oil
- 1 tsp cumin
- 1 tsp paprika
- Salt and pepper to taste

Directions

1. In a large pot, heat the olive oil over medium heat.
2. Add the garlic and onion and sauté until softened.
3. Add the carrot and cook for a few more minutes.
4. Stir in the cumin and paprika and cook for another minute.
5. Add the lentils and vegetable broth.
6. Bring to a boil, then reduce the heat and simmer for 25-30 minutes, or until the lentils are tender.
7. Add the spinach and cook for another 5 minutes.
8. Season with salt and pepper to taste and serve hot.

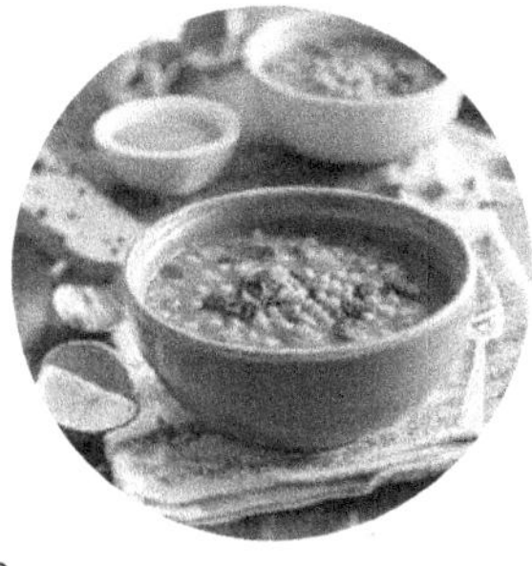

Ingredient Tips:

- Lentils: High in protein and fiber, making them excellent for managing blood sugar levels.
- Spinach: Provides fiber and essential nutrients for blood sugar control.

Broccoli and Cauliflower Soup

A creamy and delicious soup made with broccoli and cauliflower, perfect for a comforting and nutritious meal.

Servings: 4 | Prep Time: 10 mins | Cook Time: 30 mins | Carbs per Serving: 12g

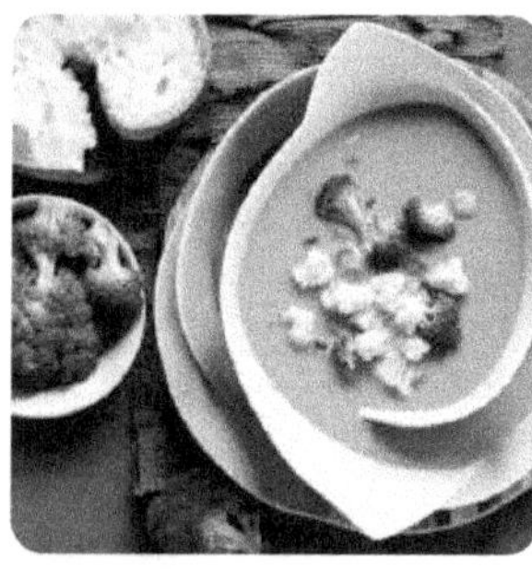

Ingredients

- 1 head broccoli, chopped
- 1 head cauliflower, chopped
- 1 onion, diced
- 2 cloves garlic, minced
- 4 cups low-sodium vegetable broth
- 1 cup unsweetened almond milk
- 1 tbsp olive oil
- Salt and pepper to taste

Directions

1. In a large pot, heat the olive oil over medium heat.
2. Add the garlic and onion and sauté until softened.
3. Add the broccoli and cauliflower and cook for a few more minutes.
4. Pour in the vegetable broth and bring to a boil.
5. Reduce heat and simmer for 20 minutes, or until the vegetables are tender.
6. Use an immersion blender to blend the soup until smooth.
7. Stir in the almond milk and season with salt and pepper to taste.
8. Serve hot.

Ingredient Tips:

- Broccoli and Cauliflower: Low in calories and high in fiber, making them great for blood sugar control.
- Almond Milk: A low-carb alternative to regular milk, keeping carbohydrate intake low.

Turkey and Vegetable Soup

A hearty soup with lean turkey and a variety of vegetables, perfect for a nutritious and balanced meal.

Servings: 4 | Prep Time: 10 mins | Cook Time: 30 mins | Carbs per serving: 10g

Ingredients

- 1 lb ground turkey
- 1 onion, diced
- 2 carrots, sliced
- 2 celery stalks, sliced
- 1 cup green beans, chopped
- 2 cloves garlic, minced
- 4 cups low-sodium chicken broth
- 1 tbsp olive oil
- Salt and pepper to taste.

Directions

1. In a large pot, heat the olive oil over medium heat.
2. Add the garlic and onion and sauté until softened.
3. Add the ground turkey and cook until browned.
4. Add the carrots, celery, and green beans and cook for a few more minutes.
5. Pour in the chicken broth and bring to a boil.
6. Reduce heat and simmer for 20 minutes.
7. Season with salt and pepper to taste and serve hot.

Ingredient Tips:

- Ground Turkey: Lean and high in protein, helping to keep you full and manage blood sugar levels.
- Green Beans: Low in calories and high in fiber, making them great for blood sugar control.

Tomato and Basil Soup

A simple and flavorful tomato soup with fresh basil, perfect for a light and satisfying meal.

Servings: 4 | Prep Time: 10 mins | Cook Time: 20 mins | Carbs per Serving: 15g

NUTRIENT CONTENT (PER SERVING):

- Calories: 120
- Total Fat: 5g
- Protein: 3g
- Carbohydrates: 15g
- Sugars: 10g
- Fiber: 5g
- Sodium: 300mg

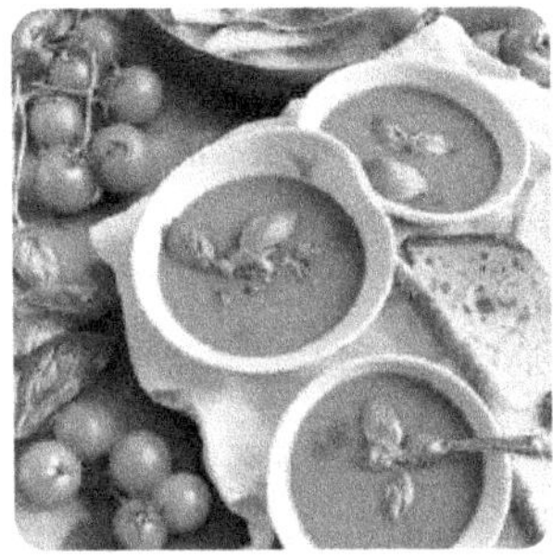

Ingredients

- 4 cups tomatoes, chopped
- 1 onion, diced
- 2 cloves garlic, minced
- 2 cups low-sodium vegetable broth
- 1 cup fresh basil, chopped
- 1 tbsp olive oil
- Salt and pepper to taste

Directions

1. In a large pot, heat the olive oil over medium heat.
2. Add the garlic and onion and sauté until softened.
3. Add the tomatoes and cook for a few more minutes.
4. Pour in the vegetable broth and bring to a boil.
5. Reduce heat and simmer for 15 minutes.
6. Use an immersion blender to blend the soup until smooth.
7. Stir in the fresh basil and season with salt and pepper to taste.
8. Serve hot.

Ingredient Tips:

- Tomatoes: Rich in vitamins and low in calories, helping to manage blood sugar levels.
- Basil: Adds flavor and nutrients without adding calories.

Butternut Squash Soup

A creamy and delicious butternut squash soup, perfect for a comforting and nutritious meal.

Servings: 4 | Prep Time: 10 mins | Cook Time: 30 mins | Carbs per serving: 20g

NUTRIENT CONTENT (PER SERVING):

- Calories: 160
- Total Fat: 6g
- Protein: 3g
- Carbohydrates: 20g
- Sugars: 8g
- Fiber: 5g
- Sodium: 300mg

Ingredients

- 1 large butternut squash, peeled and cubed
- 1 onion, diced
- 2 cloves garlic, minced
- 4 cups low-sodium vegetable broth
- 1 cup unsweetened almond milk
- 1 tbsp olive oil
- Salt and pepper to taste

Directions

1. In a large pot, heat the olive oil over medium heat.
2. Add the garlic and onion and sauté until softened.
3. Add the butternut squash and cook for a few more minutes.
4. Pour in the vegetable broth and bring to a boil.
5. Reduce heat and simmer for 20 minutes, or until the squash is tender.
6. Use an immersion blender to blend the soup until smooth.
7. Stir in the almond milk and season with salt and pepper to taste.
8. Serve hot.

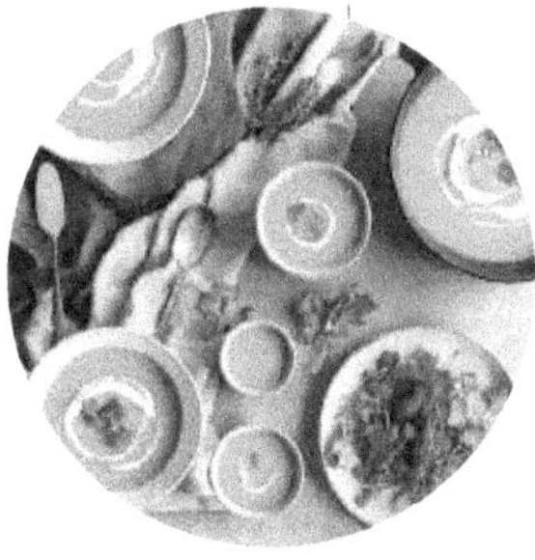

Ingredient Tips:

- Butternut Squash: High in vitamins and fiber, making it great for blood sugar control.
- Almond Milk: A low-carb alternative to regular milk, keeping carbohydrate intake low.

Mushroom and Barley Soup

A hearty and flavorful mushroom and barley soup, perfect for a nutritious and filling meal.

Servings: 4 | Prep Time: 10 mins | Cook Time: 40 mins | Carbs per Serving: 25g

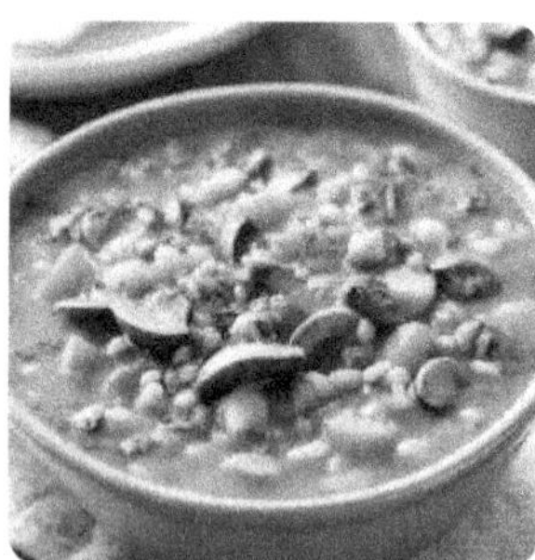

Ingredients

- 1 cup mushrooms, sliced
- 1 onion, diced
- 2 carrots, sliced
- 2 cloves garlic, minced
- 1/2 cup barley
- 4 cups low-sodium vegetable broth
- 1 tbsp olive oil
- Salt and pepper to taste

Directions

1. In a large pot, heat the olive oil over medium heat.
2. Add the garlic and onion and sauté until softened.
3. Add the mushrooms and cook until they release their juices.
4. Add the carrots and cook for a few more minutes.
5. Stir in the barley and vegetable broth.
6. Bring to a boil, then reduce the heat and simmer for 30 minutes, or until the barley is tender.
7. Season with salt and pepper to taste and serve hot.

Ingredient Tips:

- Mushrooms: Low in calories and high in nutrients, making them great for blood sugar control.
- Barley: A whole grain that provides fiber and nutrients, helping to manage blood sugar levels.

Split Pea Soup

A hearty and protein-packed split pea soup, perfect for a comforting and nutritious meal.

Servings: 4   Prep Time: 10 mins | Cook Time: 40 mins | Carbs per serving: 30g

Ingredients

- 1 cup dried split peas, rinsed
- 1 onion, diced
- 2 carrots, sliced
- 2 celery stalks, sliced
- 2 cloves garlic, minced
- 4 cups low-sodium vegetable broth
- 1 tbsp olive oil
- Salt and pepper to taste

Directions

1. In a large pot, heat the olive oil over medium heat.
2. Add the garlic and onion and sauté until softened.
3. Add the carrots and celery and cook for a few more minutes.
4. Add the split peas and vegetable broth.
5. Bring to a boil, then reduce the heat and simmer for 30-40 minutes, or until the peas are tender.
6. Season with salt and pepper to taste and serve hot.

Ingredient Tips:

- Split Peas: High in protein and fiber, making them excellent for managing blood sugar levels.
- Carrots and Celery: Provide fiber and essential nutrients for blood sugar control.

Cauliflower and Leek Soup

A creamy and delicious cauliflower and leek soup, perfect for a comforting and nutritious meal.

Servings: 4 | Prep Time: 10 mins | Cook Time: 30 mins | Carbs per Serving: 15g

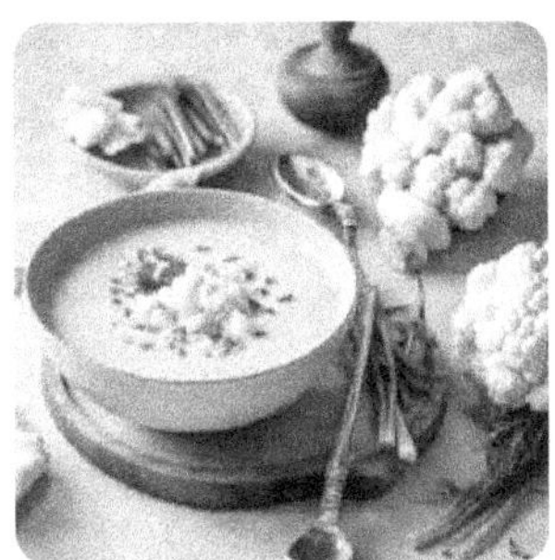

Ingredients

- 1 head cauliflower, chopped
- 2 leeks, sliced
- 1 onion, diced
- 2 cloves garlic, minced
- 4 cups low-sodium vegetable broth
- 1 cup unsweetened almond milk
- 1 tbsp olive oil
- Salt and pepper to taste

Directions

1. In a large pot, heat the olive oil over medium heat.
2. Add the garlic, onion, and leeks and sauté until softened.
3. Add the cauliflower and cook for a few more minutes.
4. Pour in the vegetable broth and bring to a boil.
5. Reduce heat and simmer for 20 minutes, or until the cauliflower is tender.
6. Use an immersion blender to blend the soup until smooth.
7. Stir in the almond milk and season with salt and pepper to taste.
8. Serve hot.

Ingredient Tips:

- Cauliflower: Low in calories and high in fiber, making it great for blood sugar control.
- Leeks: Provide flavor and nutrients without adding many calories.

Turkey Meatball Soup

A hearty and flavorful turkey meatball soup with vegetables, perfect for a nutritious and balanced meal.

Servings: 4 | Prep Time: 15 mins | Cook Time: 30 mins | Carbs per serving: 20g

Ingredients

- 1 lb ground turkey
- 1/4 cup breadcrumbs (whole grain)
- 1 egg
- 1/4 cup parmesan cheese, grated
- 1 onion, diced
- 2 carrots, sliced
- 2 celery stalks, sliced
- 4 cups low-sodium chicken broth
- 1 tbsp olive oil
- Salt and pepper to taste

Directions

1. In a bowl, mix the ground turkey, breadcrumbs, egg, parmesan cheese, salt, and pepper.
2. Form the mixture into small meatballs.
3. In a large pot, heat the olive oil over medium heat.
4. Add the garlic and onion and sauté until softened.
5. Add the carrots and celery and cook for a few more minutes.
6. Pour in the chicken broth and bring to a boil.
7. Reduce heat and simmer for 20 minutes.
8. Add the meatballs and cook for another 10 minutes, or until the meatballs are cooked through.
9. Season with salt and pepper to taste and serve hot.

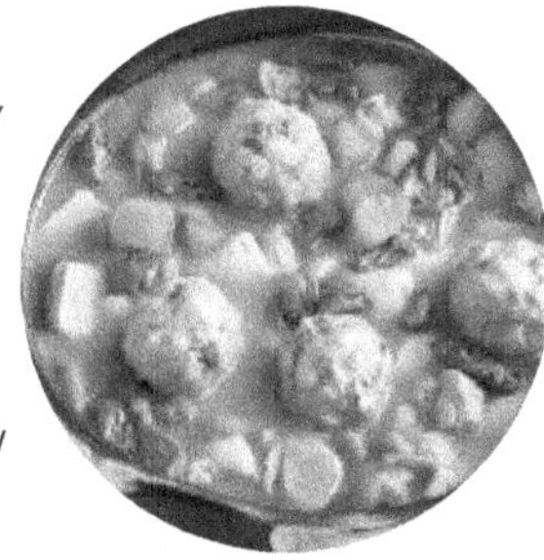

Ingredient Tips:

- Ground Turkey: Lean and high in protein, helping to keep you full and manage blood sugar levels.
- Whole Grain Breadcrumbs: Provide fiber and nutrients, making them a healthier choice.

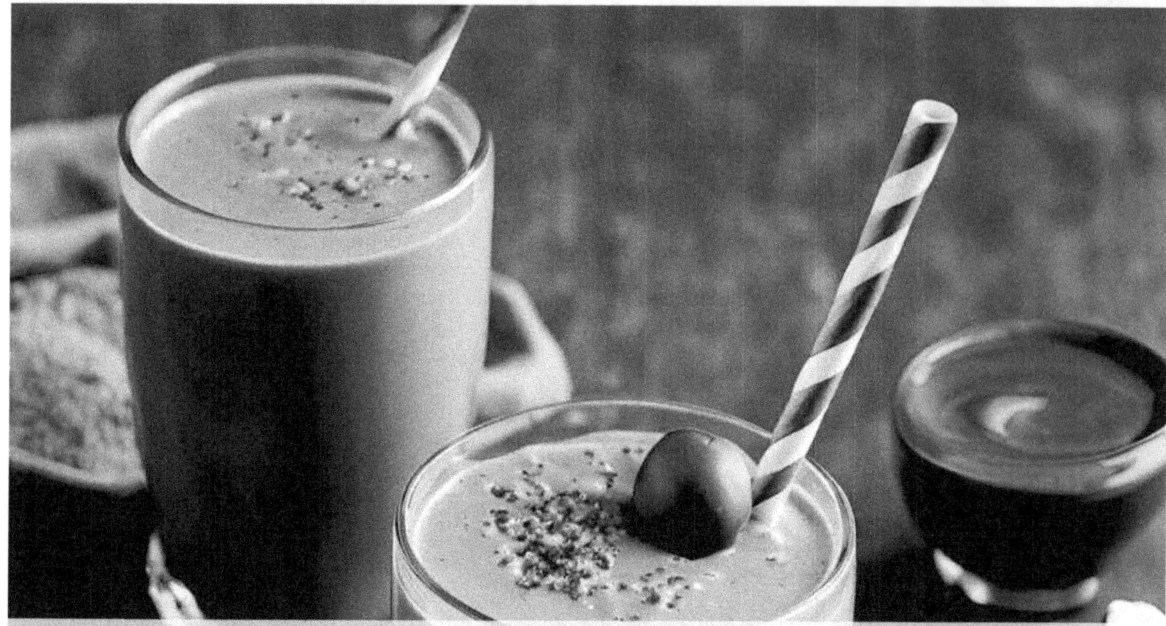

Chapter Sixteen

Smoothie Recipes

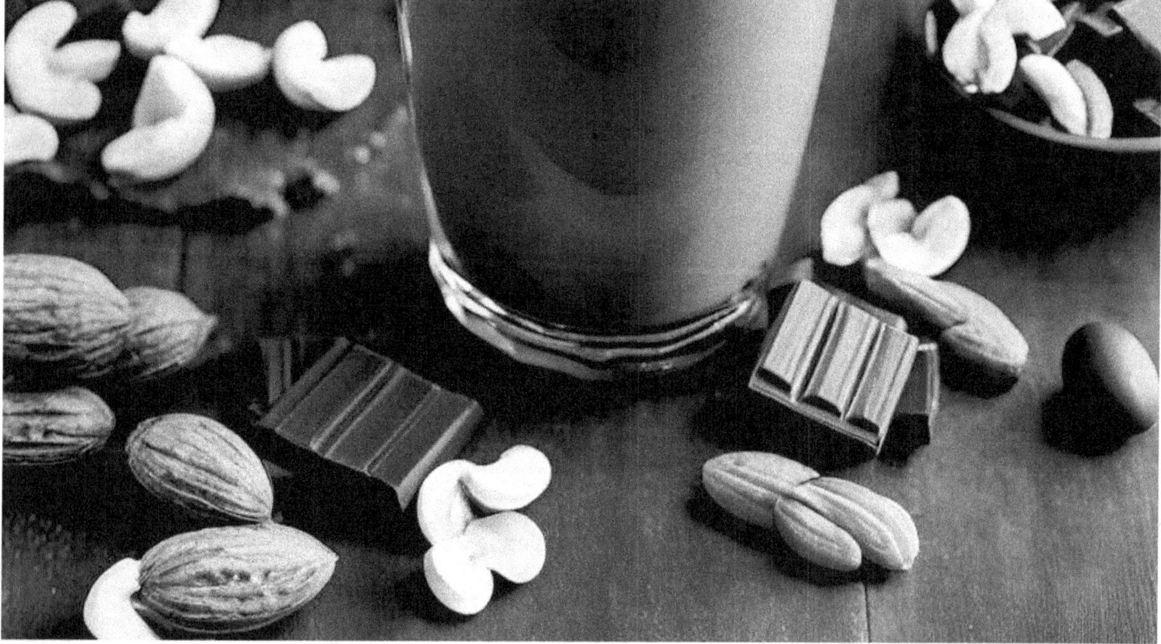

Berry Spinach Protein Smoothie

: A refreshing smoothie packed with protein, fiber, and antioxidants from berries and spinach.

Servings: 1 | Prep Time: 5 mins | Cook Time: 0 mins | Carbs per Serving: 15g

NUTRIENT CONTENT (PER SERVING):

- Calories: 200
- Total Fat: 10g
- Protein: 20g
- Carbohydrates: 15g
- Sugars: 7g
- Fiber: 7g
- Sodium: 150mg

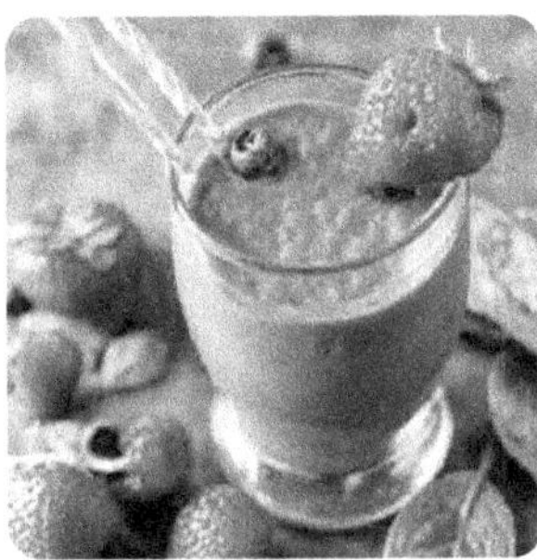

Ingredients

- 1 cup unsweetened almond milk
- 1 cup fresh spinach
- 1/2 cup mixed berries (strawberries, blueberries, raspberries)
- 1/4 avocado
- 1 scoop unflavored protein powder
- 1 tbsp chia seeds
-

Directions

1. Combine all ingredients in a blender.
2. Blend until smooth and creamy.
3. Pour into a glass and serve immediately.

Ingredient Tips:

- Mixed Berries: Low glycemic index, high in antioxidants, helping to manage blood sugar levels.
- Spinach: Rich in fiber and essential nutrients, aiding in glucose control.

Green Avocado Smoothie

A creamy and nutrient-dense smoothie with avocado, spinach, and a hint of lemon.

Servings: 1 | Prep Time: 5 mins | Cook Time: 0 mins | Carbs per serving: 12g

NUTRIENT CONTENT (PER SERVING):

- Calories: 220
- Total Fat: 15g
- Protein: 6g
- Carbohydrates: 12g
- Sugars: 2g
- Fiber: 8g
- Sodium: 90mg

Ingredients

- 1 cup unsweetened almond milk
- 1/2 avocado
- 1 cup fresh spinach
- 1/2 cucumber, chopped
- Juice of 1/2 lemon
- 1 tbsp flaxseeds

Directions

1. Add all ingredients to a blender.
2. Blend until smooth.
3. Pour into a glass and enjoy.

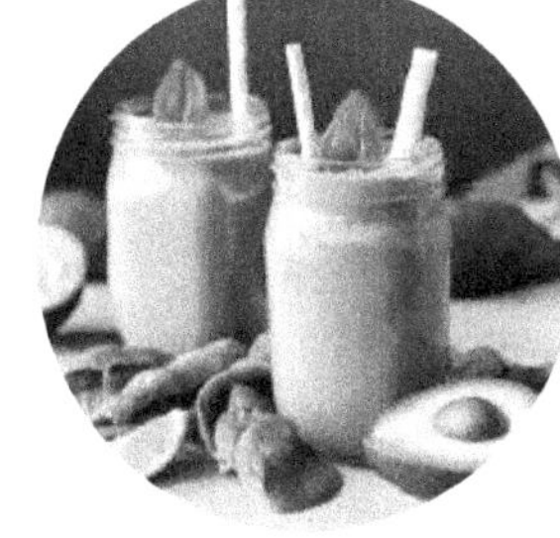

Ingredient Tips:

- Avocado: Provides healthy fats and fiber, helping to keep blood sugar levels steady.
- Cucumber: Low in calories and high in water content, promoting hydration.

Peanut Butter Banana Smoothie

A deliciously creamy smoothie with peanut butter and banana, perfect for a protein-packed breakfast.

Servings: 1 | Prep Time: 5 mins | Cook Time: 0 mins | Carbs per Serving: 20g

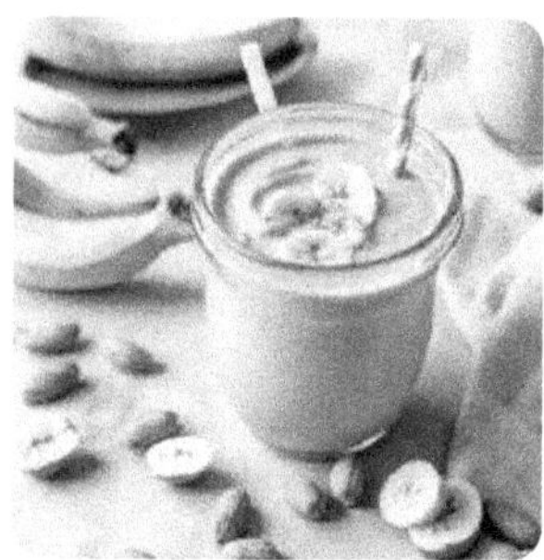

Ingredients

- 1 cup unsweetened almond milk
- 1/2 banana
- 1 tbsp natural peanut butter
- 1 scoop unflavored protein powder
- 1 tbsp chia seeds.

Directions

1. Place all ingredients in a blender.
2. Blend until smooth.
3. Pour into a glass and serve immediately.

Ingredient Tips:

- Banana: Provides natural sweetness and potassium, but use in moderation due to higher glycemic index.
- Peanut Butter: Adds protein and healthy fats, aiding in satiety and glucose control.

Blueberry Almond Smoothie

A delightful smoothie with the rich flavors of blueberries and almonds, perfect for a quick energy boost.

Servings: 1   Prep Time: 5 mins | Cook Time: 0 mins | Carbs per serving: 18g

Ingredients

- 1 cup unsweetened almond milk
- 1/2 cup fresh or frozen blueberries
- 1 tbsp almond butter
- 1 scoop unflavored protein powder
- 1 tbsp chia seeds

Directions

1. Add all ingredients to a blender.
2. Blend until smooth.
3. Pour into a glass and enjoy.

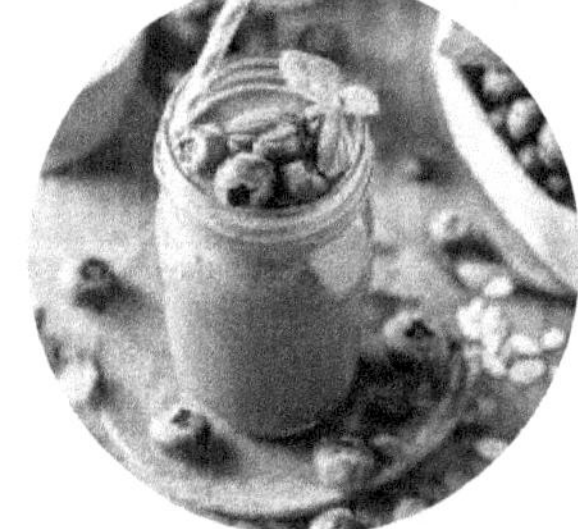

Ingredient Tips:

- Blueberries: Low glycemic index, high in antioxidants, beneficial for blood sugar control.
- Almond Butter: Provides healthy fats and protein, aiding in satiety.

Tropical Green Smoothie

A refreshing tropical smoothie with a mix of greens and tropical fruits for a balanced and nutritious drink.

Servings: 1 | Prep Time: 5 mins | Cook Time: 0 mins | Carbs per Serving: 22g

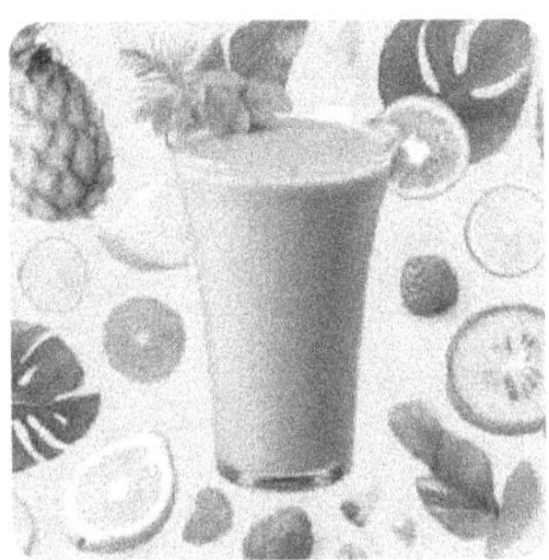

Ingredients

- 1 cup unsweetened coconut milk
- 1/2 cup pineapple chunks
- 1/2 cup mango chunks
- 1 cup fresh spinach
- 1 tbsp chia seeds

Directions

1. Place all ingredients in a blender.
2. Blend until smooth.
3. Pour into a glass and serve immediately.

Ingredient Tips:

- Pineapple and Mango: Provide natural sweetness and essential vitamins, but should be consumed in moderation.
- Coconut Milk: Adds healthy fats, enhancing satiety.

Spinach and Kiwi Smoothie

A unique and refreshing smoothie with the tangy flavor of kiwi and the nutritional benefits of spinach.

Servings: 1 | Prep Time: 5 mins | Cook Time: 0 mins | Carbs per serving: 15g

Ingredients

- 1 cup unsweetened almond milk
- 1 kiwi, peeled and sliced
- 1 cup fresh spinach
- 1/2 avocado
- 1 tbsp flaxseeds

Directions

1. Add all ingredients to a blender.
2. Blend until smooth.
3. Pour into a glass and enjoy.

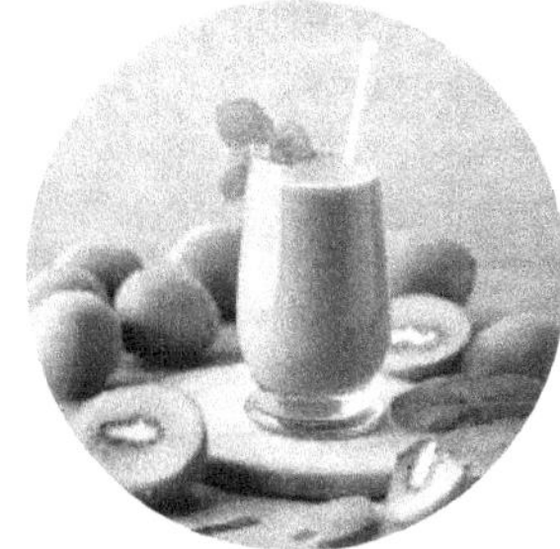

Ingredient Tips:

- Kiwi: Low glycemic index, high in vitamin C, aiding in blood sugar control.
- Flaxseeds: Provide fiber and healthy fats, beneficial for glucose management.

Cucumber Mint Smoothie

A refreshing and hydrating smoothie with the cooling flavors of cucumber and mint.

<table>
<tr><td>NUTRIENT CONTENT (PER SERVING):</td></tr>
</table>

NUTRIENT CONTENT (PER SERVING):

- Calories: 150
- Total Fat: 8g
- Protein: 4g
- Carbohydrates: 10g
- Sugars: 3g
- Fiber: 5g
- Sodium: 60mg

Servings: 1 | Prep Time: 5 mins | Cook Time: 0 mins | Carbs per Serving: 10g

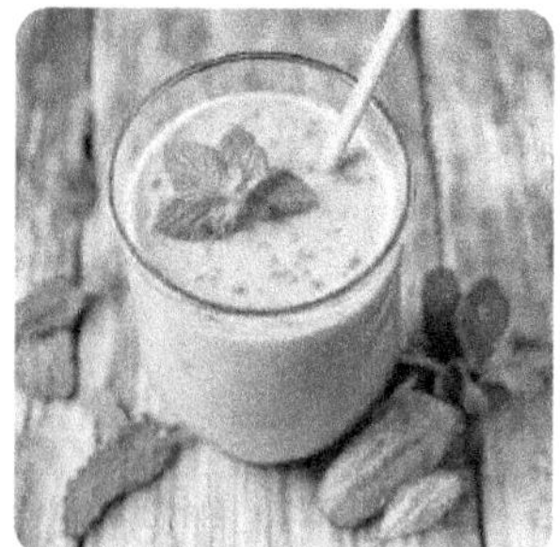

Ingredients

- 1 cup unsweetened coconut water
- 1/2 cucumber, chopped
- 1/4 avocado
- 1/4 cup fresh mint leaves
- Juice of 1/2 lime
- 1 tbsp chia seeds

Directions

1. Place all ingredients in a blender.
2. Blend until smooth.
3. Pour into a glass and serve immediately.

Ingredient Tips:

- Cucumber: Low in calories and high in water content, promoting hydration.
- Mint: Adds flavor without extra sugar or calories.

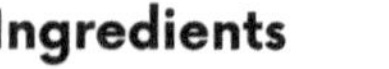

Chocolate Peanut Butter Smoothie

A rich and satisfying smoothie with the classic combination of chocolate and peanut butter.

NUTRIENT CONTENT (PER SERVING):

- Calories: 220
- Total Fat: 14g
- Protein: 20g
- Carbohydrates: 12g
- Sugars: 4g
- Fiber: 6g
- Sodium: 160mg

Servings: 1 | Prep Time: 5 mins | Cook Time: 0 mins | Carbs per serving: 15g

Ingredients

- 1 cup unsweetened almond milk
- 1 tbsp natural peanut butter
- 1 tbsp cocoa powder (unsweetened)
- 1 scoop unflavored protein powder
- 1 tbsp chia seeds

Directions

1. Add all ingredients to a blender.
2. Blend until smooth.
3. Pour into a glass and enjoy.

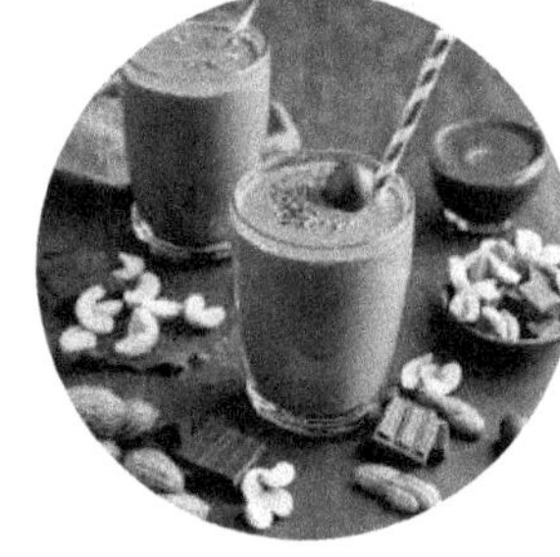

Ingredient Tips:

- Cocoa Powder: Provides a rich chocolate flavor without added sugar.
- Peanut Butter: Adds protein and healthy fats, aiding in satiety.

Strawberry Basil Smoothie

A refreshing and unique smoothie with the flavors of fresh strawberries and basil.

Servings: 1 | Prep Time: 5 mins | Cook Time: 0 mins | Carbs per Serving: 15g

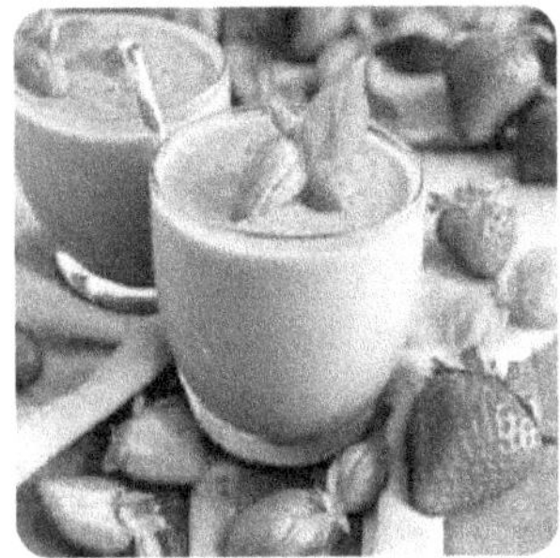

Ingredients

- 1 cup unsweetened almond milk
- 1/2 cup fresh strawberries
- 1/4 avocado
- 1/4 cup fresh basil leaves
- 1 tbsp chia seeds

Directions

1. Place all ingredients in a blender.
2. Blend until smooth.
3. Pour into a glass and serve immediately.

Ingredient Tips:

- Strawberries: Low glycemic index, high in antioxidants and vitamin C.
- Basil: Adds a unique flavor without extra sugar or calories.

Pumpkin Spice Smoothie

A seasonal favorite with the flavors of pumpkin and warm spices, perfect for a nutritious treat.

Servings: 1   Prep Time: 5 mins | Cook Time: 0 mins | Carbs per serving: 15g

Ingredients

- 1 cup unsweetened almond milk
- 1/2 cup pumpkin puree
- 1/2 banana
- 1/2 tsp cinnamon
- 1/4 tsp nutmeg
- 1 scoop unflavored protein powder
- 1 tbsp chia seeds.

Directions

1. Add all ingredients to a blender.
2. Blend until smooth.
3. Pour into a glass and enjoy.

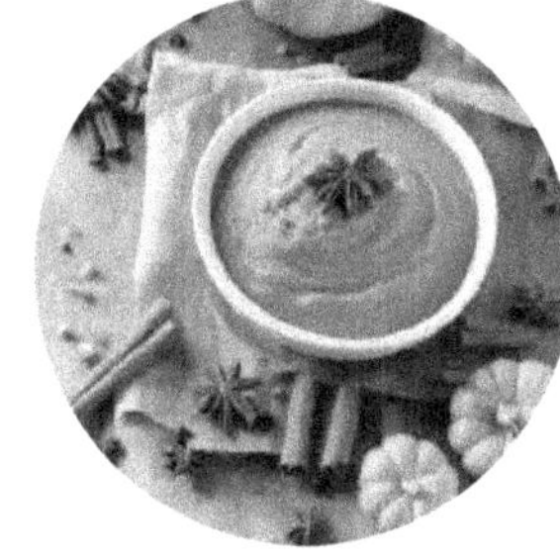

Ingredient Tips:

- Pumpkin: High in fiber and vitamins, with a moderate glycemic index.
- Spices: Add flavor and potential anti-inflammatory benefits without extra calories.

Conclusion

As you close the final chapter of "The Complete Diabetic Cookbook & Meal Plan for the Newly Diagnosed," take a moment to reflect on the journey you've embarked upon. This book isn't just a collection of recipes and meal plans; it's a guide designed to help you navigate the complexities of living with diabetes with confidence and joy.

When you first received your diagnosis, you might have felt a whirlwind of emotions—confusion, fear, maybe even a bit of anger. That's completely normal. In Part One, we delved into the essence of diabetes, unraveling its mysteries and busting common myths. You learned about the science behind the condition and why our modern diets often fall short of supporting our health. This section was all about building a solid foundation of knowledge, arming you with the information you need to make informed decisions.

Remember the chapter on "Healthy Kitchen for Diabetes Management"? Setting up a kitchen that supports your health goals is a crucial step. The tips and strategies shared there are meant to make your cooking experience enjoyable and stress-free. Your kitchen is now a sanctuary where you can create meals that nourish your body and soul.

Moving into Part Two, we crafted a four-week meal plan tailored to ease you into a new way of eating. Week by week, you were introduced to delicious, balanced meals designed to keep your blood sugar levels stable and your taste buds satisfied. The grocery shopping lists provided a roadmap, making your trips to the store efficient and purposeful.

As you followed the meal plan, you might have discovered new favorite dishes and perhaps even a newfound love for cooking. The routine of planning, shopping, and preparing meals can be a source of comfort and control, transforming what once seemed like a daunting task into an empowering daily ritual.

Part Three was where the magic truly happened—the recipes. From hearty breakfasts to delightful desserts, this section was crafted to show you that managing diabetes doesn't mean sacrificing flavor or variety. You explored a world of culinary possibilities, from vibrant salads and savory soups to satisfying mains and sweet treats. Each recipe was designed with care, keeping your health and happiness at the forefront.

Think about the first time you tried one of the breakfast recipes, or the satisfaction of cooking a wholesome dinner that everyone at the table enjoyed. Each meal is a step toward better health, each recipe a tool to help you live your best life.

Your Path Forward

Now, as you stand at the end of this book, remember that this isn't the end of your journey—it's just the beginning. The knowledge, plans, and recipes within these pages are here to support you every step of the way. Keep experimenting with new dishes, continue to plan your meals, and don't be afraid to revisit earlier chapters when you need a refresher.

Your health journey is uniquely yours, and it's filled with opportunities for growth, learning, and joy. Embrace the changes, celebrate your successes, and be kind to yourself on the tough days. You've got the tools, the knowledge, and the recipes to thrive.

Thank you for allowing this book to be a part of your journey. May your path be filled with delicious meals, vibrant health, and endless possibilities. Here's to a future where diabetes is a part of your life story—but not the defining chapter.

With warmth and encouragement,

Alina

Appendix 1: The 2024 Dirty Dozen™ and Clean Fifteen™

The Dirty Dozen and the Clean Fifteen™ refer to lists compiled by the Environmental Working Group (EWG), an organization dedicated to environmental health. They analyze data from the USDA and FDA regarding pesticide residues in commercial crops. These lists help consumers make informed choices about buying organic versus conventional produce based on pesticide levels.

The Dirty Dozen includes fruits and vegetables with the highest pesticide loads, while the Clean Fifteen™ comprises produce with lower pesticide residues. It's essential to note that even items on the Clean Fifteen™ may still have pesticide residues, so thorough washing is advised.

Since these lists are updated annually, it's crucial to check the latest version before grocery shopping.
Visit www.ewg.org/FoodNews for the most recent lists and a comprehensive guide to pesticides in produce.

DIRTY DOZEN™	CLEAN FIFTEEN™
◯ Strawberries	◯ Carrots
◯ Spinach	◯ Sweet Potatoes
◯ Kale, collard & mustard greens	◯ Mangoes
◯ Grapes	◯ Mushrooms
◯ Peaches	◯ Watermelon
◯ Pears	◯ Cabbage
◯ Nectarines	◯ Kiwi
◯ Apples	◯ Honeydew melon
◯ Bell & hot Peppers	◯ Asparagus
◯ Cherries	◯ Sweet peas (frozen)
◯ Blueberries	◯ Papaya*
◯ Green Beans	◯ Onions
	◯ Pineapple
	◯ Sweet corn*
	◯ Avocados

Appendix 2: Measurement Conversions

Volume Equivalents (Liquid)

US STANDARD	US STANDARD (OUNCES)	METRIC (APPROXIMATE)
2 tablespoons	1 fl. oz.	30 mL
¼ cup	2 fl. oz.	60 mL
½ cup	4 fl. oz.	120 mL
1 cup	8 fl. oz.	240 mL
1½ cups	12 fl. oz.	355 mL
2 cups or 1 pint	16 fl. oz.	475 mL
4 cups or 1 quart	32 fl. oz.	1 L
1 gallon	128 fl. oz.	4 L

Volume Equivalents (Dry)

US STANDARD	METRIC (APPROXIMATE)
⅛ teaspoon	0.5 mL
¼ teaspoon	1 mL
½ teaspoon	2 mL
¾ teaspoon	4 mL
1 teaspoon	5 mL
1 tablespoon	15 mL
¼ cup	59 mL
⅓ cup	79 mL
½ cup	118 mL
⅔ cup	156 mL
¾ cup	177 mL
1 cup	235 mL
2 cups or 1 pint	475 mL
3 cups	700 mL
4 cups or 1 quart	1 L

Oven Temperatures

FAHRENHEIT	CELSIUS (APPROXIMATE)
250°F	120°C
300°F	150°C
325°F	165°C
350°F	180°C
375°F	190°C
400°F	200°C
425°F	220°C
450°F	230°C

Weight Equivalents

FAHRENHEIT	CELSIUS (APPROXIMATE)
½ ounce	15g
1 ounce	30g
2 ounces	60g
4 ounces	115g
8 ounces	225g
12 ounces	340g
16 ounces or 1 pound	455g

Appendix 3: Carb Content of Foods

FRUITS

Food	Serving size	Carbs (grams)
Avocado	½ cup	8
Watermelon, diced	1 cup	11
Cantaloupe, diced	1 cup	13
Blackberries	1 cup	15
Cherries	12	15
Grapes	15	15
Nectarine, medium	1	15
Orange, medium	1	15
Raspberries	1 cup	15
Strawberries, sliced	1 cup	15
Blueberries	1 cup	18
Apple, small	1	21
Banana, 6 inches	1	23

CONDIMENTS

Food	Serving size	Carbs (grams)
Ketchup	1 tablespoon	4
White sugar	1 tablespoon	13
Jam and jelly	1 tablespoon	15
Honey	1 tablespoon	17

SNACKS AND BAKED GOODS

Food	Serving size	Carbs (grams)
Saltine crackers	5	11
Melba toast	4	15
Popcorn, air popped	3 cups	15
Pretzels, small	30	15
Tortilla chips	10 to 15	20
Donut, plain	1	25
Potato chips	30	33

VEGETABLES, STARCHY

Food	Serving size	Carbs (grams)
Peas, cooked	½ cup	10
Parsnips, cooked	½ cup	12
Corn, cooked	½ cup	15
Butternut squash	1 cup	16
Potato, mashed with milk	½ cup	17
Sweet potatoes or yams, baked without skin	1 medium	25
Potato, medium, baked with skin	1 medium	30

Appendix 3: Carb Content of Foods

BEANS, GRAINS AND PASTA		
Food	Serving size	Carbs (grams)
Tortilla, corn, 7 inches	1	11
Bread, white or whole wheat	1 slice	12 to 20
Oatmeal, quick, cooked	½ cup	13
Beans, legumes and lentils	½ cup	15 to 20
Pasta, cooked	½ cup	15 to 20
Hamburger or hotdog bun	1	15 to 30
Rice, white or brown, cooked	½ cup	22
English muffin, plain	1	25
Bagel, medium	½	25
Pita bread, 7 inches, white	1	35

DAIRY PRODUCTS AND MILK ALTERNATIVES		
Food	Serving size	Carbs (grams)
Milk	1 cup	12
Yogurt, plain	¾ cup	13
Soy milk, plain	1 cup	15
Yogurt, flavoured	1/3 cup	15
Rice milk, plain	1 cup	26

Appendix 4: Recipe Index

A

- Almond Flour Cookies, 82
- Almond Flour Pancakes with Greek Yogurt, 59
- Apple and Walnut Salad, 86
- Avocado & Chickpea Breakfast Salad, 56
- Avocado and Egg Toast, 50
- Avocado Chicken Salad, 106
- Avocado Chocolate Mousse, 81
- Avocado Deviled Eggs, 88

B

- Baked Chicken with Brussels Sprouts, 74, 108
- Baked Cod with Lemon and Asparagus, 71
- Baked Cod with Spinach & Tomatoes, 118
- Baked Cod with Tomatoes and Olives, 79
- Baked Eggplant with Tahini, 103
- Baked Pears with Cinnamon, 86
- Baked Salmon with Asparagus, 61
- Baked Salmon with Avocado Salsa, 70
- Baked Zucchini Fries, 101
- Bean and Corn Salad, 98
- Beef and Apple Skillet, 115
- Beef and Broccoli Stir-Fry, 111
- Beef and Cauliflower Rice Bowl, 113
- Beef and Lentil Stew, 112
- Beef and Vegetable Skewers, 71
- Beef, Pork & Lamb Recipes, 110
- Berry and Spinach Smoothie, 83
- Berry Spinach Protein Smoothie, 129
- Blueberry Almond Crisp, 84, 87
- Blueberry Almond Smoothie, 130
- Breakfast Recipes, 49
- Broccoli and Cauliflower Soup, 124
- Butternut Squash Soup, 125

C

- Caprese Skewers, 91
- Cauliflower and Leek Soup, 127
- Cauliflower Rice and Egg Bowl, 55
- Cauliflower Rice and Shrimp Stir-Fry, 66
- Cauliflower Rice with Herbs, 101
- Chia Seed Pudding, 81
- Chia Seed Pudding with Nuts, 55
- Chicken & Turkey Options Recipes, 105
- Chicken and Broccoli Stir-Fry, 66, 78
- Chicken and Lentil Soup, 107
- Chicken and Vegetable Curry, 73
- Chicken and Vegetable Skewers, 108
- Chicken and Vegetable Soup, 123
- Chicken Lettuce Wraps, 109
- Chickpea and Spinach Curry, 65
- Chickpea and Spinach Salad, 96
- Chickpea and Vegetable Stir-Fry, 62
- Chocolate Peanut Butter Smoothie, 132
- Coconut and Almond Energy Balls, 83, 84
- Cottage Cheese and Veggie Bowl, 53,
- Cucumber and Hummus Bites, 88
- Cucumber and Tomato Salad, 103
- Cucumber Mint Smoothie, 132

D

- Desserts Recipes, 80
- Dinner Recipes, 69

E

- Edamame with Sea Salt, 92
- Egg and Asparagus Salad, 98
- Egg and Avocado Breakfast Bowl, 58
- Egg and Veggie Breakfast Muffins, 59
- Eggplant Parmesan, 76

F

- Fish and Seafood Recipes, 116

G

- Garlic Butter Shrimp and Asparagus,   119
- Garlic Green Beans,   102
- Greek Yogurt and Cucumber Salad, 96
- Greek Yogurt and Veggie Dip, 89
- Greek Yogurt Parfait, 82
- Greek Yogurt with Nuts and Seeds, 51
- Green Avocado Smoothie, 129
- Grilled Chicken and Avocado Salad, 63
- Grilled Chicken and Spinach Salad, 94
- Grilled Chicken with Quinoa and Spinach, 70
- Grilled Salmon with Avocado Salsa, 117
- Grilled Shrimp Tacos with Avocado, 75
- Guacamole with Bell Pepper Slices, 92

L

- Lamb and Quinoa Salad, 113
- Lamb and Vegetable Kebabs, 114
- Lamb Chops with Roasted Vegetables, 112
- Lemon Garlic Butter Fish, 121
- Lemon Herb Baked Tilapia, 120
- Lemon Herb Chicken Breast, 106
- Lemon Herb Grilled Chicken, 77
- Lentil and Spinach Soup, 123
- Lentil and Tomato Salad, 94
- Lentil and Vegetable Soup, 64
- Lentil and Vegetable Stew, 67, 74
- Lentil and Veggie Lettuce Wraps, 90
- Lentil and Veggie Stir-Fry, 57
- Lunch Recipes , 60

M

- Mushroom and Barley Soup, 126
- Mushroom and Spinach Breakfast Wrap, 53

P

- Peanut Butter Banana Smoothie, 130
- Pork and Apple Skillet, 115
- Pork and Cabbage Stir-Fry, 114
- Pork Tenderloin with Spinach,   111
- Pumpkin Protein Bars, 87
- Pumpkin Spice Smoothie, 133

Q

- Quinoa and Black Bean Salad, 63
- Quinoa and Black Bean Stuffed Zucchini, 79
- Quinoa and Kale Salad, 95
- Quinoa Breakfast Bowl, 57

R

- Roasted Asparagus with Lemon and Parmesan, 102
- Roasted Brussels Sprouts with Almonds, 100
- Roasted Carrot and Lentil Salad, 104

S

- Salads and Sides Recipes, 93
- Salmon and Quinoa Salad, 120
- Salmon and Spinach Frittata, 56
- Salmon with Asparagus and Lemon, 78
- Seared Scallops with Spinach and Mushrooms, 119
- Shrimp and Avocado Salad, 97
- Shrimp and Vegetable Stir-Fry, 72, 117
- Smoked Salmon and Avocado Plate, 52
- Smoked Salmon and Avocado Toast, 58
- Smoothie Recipes, 128
- Snacks and Appetizers Recipes, 85
- Soup Recipes, 122
- Spaghetti Squash with Tomato and Basil, 77
- Spiced Nuts, 90
- Spicy Shrimp with Cauliflower Rice, 121
- Spinach & Feta Stuffed Mushrooms, 91
- Spinach and Chicken Stuffed Peppers, 107
- Spinach and Feta Scramble, 37, 43, 47, 50
- Spinach and Feta Stuffed Peppers, 61
- Spinach and Kiwi Smoothie, 131
- Spinach and Mushroom Sauté, 100
- Split Pea Soup, 126
- Strawberry Basil Smoothie, 133
- Stuffed Bell Peppers with Ground Turkey, 75
- Stuffed Bell Peppers with Quinoa, 104
-

T

- Tofu and Vegetable Stir-Fry, 67, 73
- Tofu Scramble with Veggies, 51
- Tomato and Basil Soup, 125
- Tropical Green Smoothie, 131
- Tuna and Avocado Salad, 62, 95, 118
- Turkey and Avocado Breakfast Sandwich, 54
- Turkey and Avocado Wrap, 68, 109
- Turkey and Berry Salad, 97
- Turkey and Cheese Roll-Ups, 89
- Turkey and Spinach Stuffed Portobello Mushrooms, 76
- Turkey and Spinach Wrap, 64
- Turkey and Vegetable Lettuce Wraps, 65
- Turkey and Vegetable Soup, 124
- Turkey Meatball Soup, 127
- Turkey Meatballs with Zucchini Noodles, 72
-

V

- Vegetarian Options Recipes, 99
- Veggie-Stuffed Omelet, 52

Z

- Zucchini Fritters, 54
- Zucchini Noodles with Pesto and Chicken, 68